Habermas, critical theory and health

The contribution of the German sociologist and philosopher Jürgen Habermas has proved seminal for attempts to understand the nature of social change in the context of global capitalism. This book provides an accessible introduction to his work and shows how his theories can be fruitfully applied to a wide range of topics in the sociology of health and illness including:

- lay health knowledge
- doctor–patient interaction
- health care decision making
- health inequalities
- new social movements in health
- health care rationing
- debating Foucault

This book will open up both new issues and new lines of empirical enquiry that will be of special interest to teachers and students of social theory and the sociology of health and illness, as well as to health care practitioners.

Graham Scambler is Reader in Sociology and the Director of the Centre for Medical Sociology, Social Theory and Health at University College London.

Habermas, critical theory and health

Edited by Graham Scambler

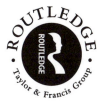

London and New York

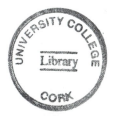

i 16612 000

First published 2001
by Routledge
11 New Fetter Lane, London EC4P 4EE

Simultaneously published in the USA and Canada
by Routledge
29 West 35th Street, New York, NY 10001

Routledge is an imprint of the Taylor & Francis Group

Typeset in Times New Roman by Taylor and Francis Books Ltd
Printed and bound in Great Britain by TJ International Ltd,
Padstow, Cornwall.

British Library Cataloguing in Publication Data
A catalogue record for this book is available from the British
Library

Library of Congress Cataloging in Publication Data
Habermas, critical theory and health/edited by Graham Scambler
Includes bibliographical data and information
1. Habermas, Jürgen. 2. Medical sociology. 3. Medicine–Philosophy.
4. Social
RA418 .H23 2001
306.4'61–dc21

ISBN 0–415–19181–5 (hbk)   00-051776
ISBN 0–415–19182–3 (pbk)

Contents

Contributors

Nicky Britten is Senior Lecturer in Medical Sociology and Director of the Concordance Unit in the Department of General Practice and Primary Care at the Guy's, King's and St Thomas' School of Medicine. Her research interests include the social aspects of drugs and medicines, prescribing and medicine taking. She has recently been awarded a senior research fellowship by the British Academy to research the sociology of doctor–patient communication about medicines.

Paul Higgs is Senior Lecturer in Sociology at University College London, where he teaches on the M.Sc in 'Sociology, Health and Health Care'. His interests include social theory and social policy, the concept of ideology and the sociology of later life. He co-edited *Modernity, Medicine and Health* (Routledge, 1998), and, with Chris Gilleard, recently published *Cultures of Ageing: Self, Citizen and the Body* (Prentice-Hall, 2000).

Ian Rees Jones is Professor of Sociology of Health and Illness at St George's Hospital Medical School, London. He is author of *Professional Power and the Need for Health Care* (Ashgate, 1999).

David Kelleher is Senior Research Fellow at London Guildhall University. For the past twenty years he has been researching and writing about how lay people understand chronic illness. He edited *Challenging Medicine* with Jonathan Gabe and Gareth Williams (Routledge, 1994), and, with Sheila Hillier, *Researching Cultural Differences in Health* (Routledge, 1996). He has used his long-time interest in Habermas to attempt to make theoretical sense of lay knowledge in some of these writings and draws on these in his chapter in this book.

Leslie Martin is currently a graduate student in the Department of Sociology at Emory University, Atlanta, USA. Her interests include urban sociology and neighbourhood activism.

Jennie Popay was Professor of Sociology and Community Health at the University of Salford and Director of the Institute for Public Health Research and Policy until November 2000, when she moved to take up a Chair in Sociology and Health Policy at the Nuffield Institute for Health, Leeds University. She has published widely in the fields of sociology of health and social policy. Her research interests include gender and class inequalities in health and the sociology of knowledge, with particular reference to the relationship between lay and professional knowledge in the field of public health. Her recent publications include the edited collections *Men, Gender Divisions and Welfare* (with Jeff Hearn and Jeanette Edwards, Routledge, 1998) and *Welfare Research: A Critical Review* (with Fiona Williams and Ann Oakley, UCL Press, 1999).

Graham Scambler is Reader in Sociology and Director of the Centre for Medical Sociology, Social Theory and Health at University College London. He teaches on the M.Sc in 'Sociology, Health and Health Care' at UCL, and his areas of interest include philosophy and social theory, coping with chronic illness and health inequalities. He has published widely in academic journals and his books include *Modernity, Medicine and Health* (co-edited with Paul Higgs, Routledge, 1998), and *Health and Social Change: A Critical Theory* (Open University Press, forthcoming).

Gareth Williams was Professor of Sociology and Deputy Director of the Public Health Research and Resource Centre at the University of Salford until 1999. He is now Professor and Director of Research in the School of Social Sciences at Cardiff University. He has published widely in academic and professional journals on subjects relating to chronic illness and disability, the relationship between lay and professional knowledge, health services and policy, and social inequalities in health. He is co-author or editor of a number of books including *Challenging Medicine* (Routledge, 1994), *Researching the People's Health* (Routledge, 1994), *Understanding Rheumatoid Arthritis* (Routledge, 1996), *Markets and Networks* (Open University Press, 1996) and *Contracting for Health* (1997).

Chapter 1

Introduction

Unfolding themes of an incomplete project

Graham Scambler

It is ironic that while Jürgen Habermas is arguably the premier social theorist of his generation, his work is probably less known and discussed, at least among his Anglo-Saxon peers, and certainly less often used or put to the test in substantive areas of inquiry, than that of numerous more transient or superficial thinkers. Undoubtedly this is in part because of the scope of his interests and his dense, heavy and discouraging writing style. It is probably due in no small measure too to his determined opposition to the – frequently faddish – excesses of postmodern texts (see Habermas, 1987a). This volume as a whole sets out to begin to make good the neglect of Habermas' work within the specialist domain of medical sociology.

It is the more specific function of this opening chapter to give an indication of the direction, unfolding, revision and current thrust of Habermas' large and wide-ranging corpus. This is no small task. Not only has Habermas contributed in depth over the years to an extraordinary variety of discussions and debates, many of his interjections straddling disciplinary boundaries, but he has constantly learned from others and modified his own positions publicly in consequence (Holub, 1991).

The strategy will be to open with a brief reminder of the origins of Habermas' work in the early critical theory of the Frankfurt School. The links between these antecedents and his own initial ventures are important. Punctuating a general and somewhat cursory review of his early work (for a far more comprehensive consideration, see McCarthy, 1978) will be a (marginally) more detailed inspection of two especially telling early analyses – namely, those concerning the 'bourgeois public sphere' (Habermas, 1989) and 'crises of legitimation' (Habermas, 1976) – which have

deservedly attracted renewed interest. The main focus of the
chapter will then switch to a fuller exposition of his later and core
theories of communicative action (Habermas, 1984, 1987) and
discourse ethics (Habermas, 1990a) and his current excursions into
the law, rights and democratic practice (Habermas, 1996).

A tradition of critical theory

The concept of 'critical theory', and even the phrase itself, have
long and vital histories, and it would be inappropriate to attribute
exclusive proprietorship to those philosophers and social theorists
pre-eminent in 'cultural critique' in Frankfurt in the inter-war years
and later, with the advent of Nazism, in California. Under the inspi-
ration of the likes of Horkheimer and Adorno, and in the 1960s in
the USA Marcuse, a flexible neo-Marxist perspective evolved,
framed in response to fascism, Stalinism and managerial capitalism
(Outhwaite, 1996).

Born in 1926, Habermas became Adorno's assistant during the
period of return to Germany after the Second World War, and later
the leading exponent of second-generation critical theory. Beilharz
(1995: 40) is not alone in observing that 'the relationship between
the two generations is a complicated matter, for to skim through the
work by, say, Adorno and Habermas is to wonder what connection
there might be at all'. Adorno, a philosopher, is associated with a
remorseless cultural pessimism, the logic of which is that 'the twentieth century and even modernity itself are long arcs of irrevocable
decline' (Beilharz, 1995: 40). Adorno's classic, *Dialectic of
Enlightenment*, written with Horkheimer during the Second World
War but published in 1947, set in the shadow of the Holocaust,
epitomizes this inexorable sense of decay (Horkheimer and Adorno,
1982).

Habermas did not share his mentors' gloom. And it was his
concept of rationality which was to differentiate his theories from
those of predecessors like Marx, Weber, Adorno and Horkheimer.
He rejected what he took to be their equation between rationality
and what Weber called *Zweckrationalit* or 'instrumental rationality'.
Instrumental rationality refers to the rationality that governs the
choice of means to given – often material – ends. Habermas was to
contrast this with 'communicative rationality', which refers to the
activity of reflecting upon our background assumptions about the
world and 'bringing our basic norms to the fore, to be questioned

and negotiated' (Braaten, 1991: 12). Instrumental rationality takes these 'background assumptions' for granted. Moreover, it is insufficient on its own, Habermas was to contend, to capture the natures of either 'cultural evolution', which is not governed by instrumental reason alone, or economic and administrative systems, which are too complex to be seen merely as its products. But if these themes were represented in his early work, they were only to be fully elaborated much later.

Early texts

Habermas' first major book was *The Structural Transformation of the Public Sphere*, which appeared in 1962 (and arose out of an 'Habilitation' thesis rejected by Adorno but supported subsequently by Abendroth at Marburg). The logic of this postdoctoral inquiry was precisely to put what Beilharz (1995: 2) calls 'an unwelcome emancipatory twist on *Dialectic of Enlightenment*'. In it Habermas seeks to trace the concept of public opinion back to its historical roots in the bourgeois public sphere emergent in eighteenth-century Europe. It was at this time, he argues, that the literate bourgeois public began to assume a political role in the evaluation of contemporary issues and, especially, of state policy. The clubs, coffee-houses and salons that sprang up from the early 1700s, supported by a growing and increasingly free press, provided a critical forum 'in which gentlemen independent of the court and other political institutions could get together on a basis of relative equality and discuss the great events of the day' (Outhwaite, 1996a: 8).

Habermas identifies as one cause of this development the enhanced salience of state policy for the growing bourgeoisie during a period of rapid expansion of trade and industry: quite apart from any resurgence of a democratic impulse, the bourgeoisie urgently required to be familiar with state policy making and to influence it whenever possible. Outhwaite (1996a: 8) suggests that this manner of explaining the advent of a bourgeois public sphere may be rather materialist, but rightly adds that the ideal of rational, informed discussion of public policy 'runs like a red thread' through Habermas' later work.

Habermas admits that this European prototype of what he later refers to as the 'public use of reason' was always compromised: he acknowledges, for example, if he arguably makes too little of, the limitations of class and gender. He also notes tendencies to commercialization, going on to chart a rapid subsequent transformation or 're-feudalization' of the public sphere. The principle of critical publicity became progressively more diluted with the expansion of the state's role (culminating in 'welfare statism') and the growth of large private concerns and of the mass media. 'Whereas the press could previously merely mediate the reasoning process of the private people who had come together in public', he stresses, 'this reasoning is now, conversely, only formed by the mass media' (Habermas, 1989: 188). The political process similarly changed: a cleavage occurred between party activists on the one hand, and an essentially inactive and passive mass electorate on the other. Public opinion was no longer a source of critical judgement, but became a social-psychological variable to be manipulated. In short, the public sphere was 'smothered through colonization by instrumental reason' (Beilharz, 1995: 57).

Outhwaite shrewdly asks if this analysis might not be seen as a 'social-scientific remake' of Horkheimer and Adorno's *Dialectic of Enlightenment*. He writes, 'just as the enlightenment critique of myth turned into another myth, the principle of the bourgeois sphere, the critical assessment of policy in terms of rational discussion oriented to a concept of the public interest, turns into what Habermas calls a manipulated public sphere in which states and corporations use "publicity" in the modern sense to secure for themselves a kind of plebiscitary acclamation' (Outhwaite, 1996a: 10). The point was made earlier however, and Outhwaite notes it too, that Habermas has proved altogether more cautious and less pessimistic than his predecessors.

Habermas has revised and extended his approach to the public sphere over the years and both his early and later works have exerted a considerable influence on current accounts of 'civil society' (see Calhoun, 1992; Habermas, 1992). A number of the pertinent issues are directly addressed in Chapter 9 of this volume.

During the 1960s Habermas published four further volumes in Germany: *On the Logic of the Social Sciences* (1990), *Theory and Practice* (1986), *Towards a Rational Society* (1986a) and *Knowledge and Human Interests* (1986b). The first of these provides an informed and innovative survey of the methods deployed by the social sciences in the mid-1960s and remains a useful resource. *Theory and Practice*, a series of studies published in 1963, has as its general focus the relationship between theory and practice in the social sciences; but most relevant here, perhaps, is Habermas' early response to Marx, which prefigures his attempt to 'reconstruct' historical materialism. Habermas distinguishes between 'work' and 'interaction', a distinction of key significance in his critical appropriation of Marxism. According to him, Marx fails both to make such a distinction and to attend adequately to interaction, and as a result reduces communicative action to instrumental action, that is, to 'the productive activity which regulates the material interchange of the human species with its natural environment' (Habermas, 1986: 169). This deficiency encourages a 'misinterpretation' of Marxism in terms of a mechanistic relationship between forces and relations of production which undermines it both as an explanatory theory and as a theory of human liberation (Outhwaite, 1996a). Habermas (1986: 169; original emphasis) writes, 'to set free the technical forces of production... is not identical with the development of moral relationships in an interaction free of domination. ... *Liberation from hunger and misery* does not necessarily converge with *liberation from servitude and degradation*; for there is no automatic developmental relation between labour and interaction.'

Towards a Rational Society was published in Germany in 1968 and, aptly, among its concerns was the student movement and the role of universities. Habermas again emphasizes the significance of the distinction between work and interaction and of the neglect of the latter. At several points he pursues the contention that the progressive 'rationalization' of society is intimately linked to the institutionalization of scientific and technological development. To the extent that science and technology permeate social institutions, old legitimations are destroyed and a 'scientization of politics' is threatened. He considers the possibility of students activating a 'new conflict zone' to challenge this 'technocratic background ideology' of depoliticization.

There are those who judge *Knowledge and Human Interests* to be the most original of Habermas' volumes to date (Rockmore, 1989). It certainly offered at its time of publication in 1968 a full and more rounded statement of earlier tendencies. In Scott's (1995: 231) succinct phrasing, Habermas espouses the thesis that the historical production of knowledge is 'structured by universal and a priori "cognitive interests" that are features of the human "species being", essential characteristics of human life. These cognitive interests ... are transcendental "knowledge-constitutive" interests that guide the search for knowledge. They are fundamental and invariant orientations to knowledge and action that are rooted in the universal conditions and circumstances of the evolution of the human species, understood as a process of "self-formation".' The concepts of work and interaction are central to this thesis, augmented by a third basic form of action, domination. This leads to the following threefold categorization. First, the natural or *empirical-analytical* sciences are governed by a 'technical' interest in the prediction and control of objectified processes: 'the facts relevant to the empirical sciences are first constituted through an *a priori* interest in the behavioural system of instrumental action' (Habermas, 1986b: 109). Second, the *historical-hermeneutic* sciences are governed by a 'practical' interest in intersubjective understanding. And third, the *critical-dialectical* sciences, like psychoanalysis and the critique of ideology, are directed to 'emancipation' from domination of what Habermas (1986b: 310) calls 'ideologically frozen relations of dependence that can in principle be transformed'. Habermas came to see this thesis of knowledge-constitute interests as problematic and in need of recasting, principally because, as a social theory of knowledge, it introduced a circularity into his position: *social* theory must provide the foundations for a theory of knowledge, but this theory of knowledge must itself provide the unassailable foundations for social theory (Scott, 1995). It was a circularity he was determined to overcome.

Legitimation Crisis (1976), or, in a more literal translation of the German original, 'Problems of Legitimation in Late Capitalism', was published in Germany in 1974. Habermas' analysis of liberal capitalism remains essentially Marxist; but in his analysis of post-liberal, advanced or late capitalism he disputes the orthodox Marxist insistence on the pre-potency of economic crisis, proposing instead a multiplicity of possible crises.

Reflecting on the enhanced salience and steering capacities of the state in late capitalism, he anticipates a number of associated 'crisis tendencies'. The state in late capitalism, he reasons, self-consciously acts to avoid dysfunctions, a strategy he terms 'reactive crisis avoidance'. Specifically, the state attempts to 'iron out' the peaks and troughs of the business cycle and to mitigate the opposition between wage labour and capital to engineer politically a 'partial class compromise'. But if the activities of the state serve to forestall economic collapse and class conflict, this is not achieved without costs.

Habermas argues that the potential economic crises faced in late capitalism, which are managed and contained by the 'political counter control' of the state, 'are not expelled from the social system, but merely displaced into other spheres' (Lawrence, 1989: 138). Thus economic crises in late capitalism may be resolved through state intervention, but only by displacing them into the political domain. In fact the state, as Sitton (1996: 154) explains, has two primary tasks: on the one hand, it has to raise and utilize taxes 'so rationally that crisis-ridden disturbances of growth can be avoided'. On the other hand, it must raise and utilize taxes in such a way that 'the need for legitimation can be satisfied as it arises'. Failure in the former results in a 'deficit in administrative rationality'; failure in the latter results in a 'deficit in legitimation'.

A deficit in legitimation, or a legitimation crisis, is the more threatening for government. Habermas, rather like Offe, maintains that state intervention directly courts a legitimation crisis in that it makes the state responsible for managing the economy: 'because the economic crisis has been intercepted and transformed into a systematic overloading of the public budget, it has put off the mantle of a natural fate of society. If governmental crisis management fails, it lags behind programmatic demands *that it has placed on itself*. The penalty for this failure is withdrawal of legitimation' (original emphasis).

Habermas is clear that an authentic legitimation of late capitalism is not possible because of the continued existence of its class structure. Even if growth without crisis occurs, the fundamental 'contradiction' of the capitalist system – 'between the social process of production and the private appropriation and use of the product' (Beetham, 1991: 166) – remains. The priorities of the system are based not on 'generalizable interests' but on the 'private goals of profit maximization'. Public policy is driven by a 'class structure that is, as usual, kept latent'. 'In the final analysis, *this class structure* is the source of the legitimation deficit' (Habermas, 1976: 2; original emphasis).

A legitimation crisis is contingent upon what Habermas calls a 'motivation crisis', namely, 'a discrepancy between the need for motives declared by the state, the educational system and the occupational system on the one hand, and the motivation supplied by the socio-cultural system on the other' (Habermas, 1976: 74–5). A motivation crisis occurs when there are changes in the socio-cultural system such that its 'output' becomes 'dysfunctional' for the state and the system of social labour. The motivations most important for late capitalism are discussed under the rubric of 'civil and familial-vocational privatism'. In more mundane terms, this refers to both the mass, diffuse loyalty associated with formal (parliamentary) democracy, and family and career orientations suitable to status competition.

The final text to be mentioned in this opening section is *Communication and the Evolution of Society* (1991), published in Germany in 1976. This is another varied volume, reflecting ongoing work on language and speech acts, psychological and moral development, and social evolution. Comment will be restricted here to the attempt to proffer a 'reconstruction' of Marx's historical materialism. Like *Legitimation Crisis*, it might be described as a contribution 'which is simultaneously for and against or beyond Marx' (Beilharz, 1995: 47).

Outhwaite (1996a: 59) suggests that Habermas' arguments are elaborations on two basic claims. The first is that the development of human society can be represented or reconstructed as a learning process; and the second is that historical materialism is, or can be reconstructed as, the best available theory of this process. As has already been noted, Habermas believes Marx concentrated too much on work and too little on interaction. He offers a reconstruction of historical materialism which accepts the primacy of the 'base' over the 'superstructure', understood in terms of 'the leading role that the economic structure assumes in social evolution' (Habermas, 1976: 143); but he insists that the base–superstructure distinction cannot account for the attainment of new forms of social integration, which can only be explained by advances at the level of communicative action which 'follow their own logic'. Thus he advocates 'the search for highly abstract principles of social organization ... which institutionalize new levels of societal learning' (Habermas, 1996: 155). 'Such principles', in Outhwaite's (1996a: 61) words, 'are embodied in moral and legal systems, grounded in socially shared world-views.'

This review of Habermas' early work has been partial, uncritical and inevitably gives only a flavour of his multiple interests and interventions through the 1960s and 1970s. For the most part the focus has been on issues which have continued to impress themselves upon him since then. In the next section, which concentrates on a considerable work of synthesis, *Theory of Communicative Action*, it will be seen how he develops, refines, reconstructs, rethinks and occasionally rejects some of his initial stances.

Although his more recent endeavours are treated here rather more fully than his early ones, there is once again space only for limited exposition.

The Theory of Communicative Action

The mammoth two-volume *Theory of Communicative Action* (1984, 1987), published in Germany in 1981, is too dense and wide-ranging to be summarized adequately here. It will suffice, however, to pick up on a number of central themes, namely, the general recasting or reconstruction of the philosophical legacy of the European Enlightenment; the linguistic kernel to the theory of communicative action; the theory of social evolution and the virtues and limitations of a Marxist perspective; the putative uncoupling of system and lifeworld in modernity; and system and lifeworld rationalization.

It seems rarely to be recognized that Habermas has been as damning of the *unreconstructed* Enlightenment project as any author now likely to attract the sobriquet 'postmodernist'; but whereas postmodernists have judged the Enlightenment project to be flawed beyond redemption, Habermas has committed himself to its necessary and compelling reconstruction. It was Kant (1970: 54) who characterized the Enlightenment as 'man's emergence from self-incurred immaturity'. The project pioneered and commended by philosophers like Kant 'consisted in their efforts to develop objective science, universal morality and law, and autonomous art according to their inner logic. At the same time, this project intended to release the cognitive potentials of each of these domains from their esoteric forms. The Enlightenment philosophers wanted to utilize this accumulation of specialized culture for the enrichment of everyday life – that is to say, for the rational organi-zation of everyday life' (Habermas, 1981: 9). The commitment to a defence of a reconstructed version of this project can be discerned throughout Habermas' corpus, increasingly from the 1970s onwards, against those he regards as agents of counter-Enlightenment, such as Nietzsche, Heidegger, Bataille and their intellectual progeny (Best and Kellner, 1991; see Habermas, 1987a).

Habermas (1984) argues that Weber's concepts of rationality and rationalization are overly restrictive and insufficiently abstract. This misled Weber in two ways. First, distracted by the extent of the vari-ation in their *contents*, he underestimated the extent to which rationality and rationalization in the different 'value spheres' – of science, morality and art – possess the same formal or procedural properties. And second, he wrongly argued that the value spheres are not only inherently irreconcilable, but become more overtly and explicitly so the further rationalization progresses. Habermas, by contrast, espouses the universality of reason, and maintains that the value spheres have come to *appear* increasingly irreconcilable mainly because of 'selective rationalization' consequent on the growth and dominance of the capitalist economy and state bureaucracy (Brand, 1990).

Habermas' defence of the notion of universal reason yields a formal or procedural concept of rationality owing much to the linguistic turn in twentieth-century Anglo-Saxon philosophy. He argues that reason can no longer be claimed to issue from the subject–object relations of the philosophy of consciousness, be it in Kantian, Hegelian or Marxian forms. Rather, it issues from the subject–subject relations of communicative action. What Brand (1990) terms Habermas' 'central intuition' is that people's use of language implies a common endeavour to attain consensus in a context in which all participants are free to contribute and have equal opportunities to do so. Language use, in short, presupposes commitment to the 'ideal speech situation', in which discourse can realize its full potential. It does not follow that the ideal speech situation is readily accomplished, but it does mean that communicative action, although always occurring in a particular cultural context, rests also on an ahistorical factor. 'This factor', Brand (1990: 11–12) elaborates, 'is found in the claim for the validity of the reasons which induce people to take their particular share in communicative action. In such claims no historical limitation is recognized since they are based on the (implicit) view that their validity should be accepted by anyone capable of judgement who is free to use it, whether in the past, present or future. The idea of rationally motivated shared understanding – and rational motivation implies the total lack of compulsion or manipulation – is built into the very reproduction of social life, or so Habermas claims. The symbolic reproduction of society is based on the "counterfactual" ideal of the "ideal speech situation", which is characterized by "communicative symmetry" and a compulsion-free consensus' (see also Scambler, 1996).

The concept of communicative action is bound up with Habermas' 'formal pragmatics', which draws on Austin's (1962) notion of speech acts, adumbrated in his earlier texts (Habermas,

1991; see also Habermas, 1998); this is explored in more depth in Chapter 4.

But what, next, of Habermas' theory of social evolution, and, more precisely, of his affinity with Marx? For Habermas, 'social evolution is seen as a learning process for the human species, a process in which the species as a whole comes to appreciate its own powers and capabilities' (Scott, 1995: 245). Unfashionably and ambitiously, he draws parallels between personal and social evolution. Against the relativist, he contends, as has been seen, that 'procedurally the canons of rationality – that is to say, the modes of reaching warranted conclusions – are the same everywhere' (Giddens, 1985: 132). This makes it possible for both individuals and cultures to be located on scales of evolutionary development, using 'cognitive adequacy' as the criterion: cognitive adequacy refers to the range and depth of the defensible validity claims available. As far as individuals are concerned, Habermas starts from Piaget's theory that there are three stages of cognitive development in children, representing a progressive expansion of their learning capacities. With reference to cultures, he maintains that there are likewise three stages of development or evolution: the 'mythical' (as found in 'primitive' societies), the 'religious-metaphysical' (as found in 'traditional' societies), and the 'post-conventional' (as found in 'modern' societies).

For Piaget the higher levels of cognitive development signify a 'decentration' of an egocentrically distorted appreciation of the world. Individuals move from a narrow preoccupation with their own immediate needs to an enlarged awareness of a world independent of themselves and the needs of others. Cultures or 'world-views', Habermas suggests, undergo an analogous process of transformation. Primitive cultures are dominated by myth: they are typically 'closed' and refractory to change. Social organization is the product of established practice rather than rational argument. Moreover, the institutional conditions for reasoned public engagement are lacking. Rationality is expanded, however, with the emergence and spread of religions like Buddhism, Hinduism, Islam and Christianity, which are broader-based than myth. Like Weber, Habermas sees religion as contributing to the rationalization of culture, culminating in modern western capitalism. But he differs from Weber in his association of rationalization with the further expansion of rationality. Modern capitalism, he argues, is characterized by postconventional cognitive domains. And postconventional cognitive forms of social organization, unlike those based on the now 'disvalued' myth of the religious-metaphysical, are based on warranted principles (Habermas, 1984: 68). This does not of course mean that Habermas is uncritical of modern capitalism, but he does see undeniable gains in the potential for human enlightenment. Schmidt (1982: 18) observes that he constructs a defence of the potential for enlightenment based on an 'enlightened suspicion of enlightenment'.

All this seems a far cry from Marx; and yet Habermas has consistently declared himself to be a Marxist, if a critical one. A convincing reconstruction of Marx's historical materialism has been a long-term goal of his (although numerous expositors have noted a progressive distancing from Marxian orthodoxy and what they see as a revised project to 'replace' rather than reconstruct historical materialism (see Rockmore, 1989)). Outhwaite (1996a: 17) suggests that Habermas' relationship to Marxism might be described as 'one of positive critique'. It will be remembered that Habermas distinguished early in his published interventions between work and interaction, charging Marx (and, even more vigorously, some Marxists), as well as Weber and his own predecessors at Frankfurt, with a fixation on the former and a fateful neglect of the latter. In the case of Marxian theory, what Habermas takes to be the reduction of interaction (or communicative action) to work (or strategic action) not only dramatically inhibits the scope of the sociological analysis of modernity, but eliminates any potential to ground a project of human liberation.

According to Sitton (1996: 168), the overriding goal of Habermas' theoretical endeavours has been to find a way of combining the two leading approaches to social theory, namely, 'the perspective that analyzes society as a meaningful whole for its participants (Verstehen theory) and the perspective that analyzes society as a system that is stabilized behind the backs of the participants (system theory)'. In Theory of Communicative Action, these two approaches resolve into, respectively, a focus on the action orientations of society's members, and a focus on how the action consequences are coordinated without necessitating the will or consciousness of the participants. And this gives rise to the celebrated distinction between the lifeworld, based on social integration, and the system, based on system integration.

The lifeworld begs easy definition, cannot be 'known' since it serves as the vehicle of all knowing. Individuals can no more step outside their lifeworld than they can their language. But, as Sitton (1996: 169) again states: 'although the lifeworld as a whole can never be placed in question, elements of the lifeworld can be and are placed in doubt. In these cases, the element is "thematized", made subject to argument as the participants attempt to re-establish their mutual definition of the situation, a prerequisite for successful cooperation.' Thus the lifeworld can be reproduced through communicative action, but not through instrumental or strategic action. The lifeworld, Habermas goes on to argue, is the medium, or 'symbolic space', within which culture, social integration and personality are sustained and reproduced (Thompson, 1984).

The system pertains to material rather than symbolic reproduction, and is characterized by strategic rather than communicative action. Habermas maintains, in neo-Parsonian fashion, that societal differentiation has produced four subsystems: the economy, the state, the public sphere and the private sphere. Moreover, there has been a fundamental 'uncoupling' between the economy and the state, which constitute the system, on the one hand, and the public and private spheres, which constitute the lifeworld, on the other. These subsystems are interdependent: each is specialized in terms of what it produces but is dependent on the others for what it does not produce. The economy produces 'money', the state 'power', the public sphere 'influence', and the private sphere 'commitment'. The products or *media* are traded between subsystems. For example, in the words of Crook *et al.* (1992: 28): 'the economy relies on the state to establish such legal economic institutions as private property and contract, on the public lifeworld to influence consumption patterns, and on the private lifeworld to provide a committed labour force, and itself sends money into each other subsystem'.

The media of the subsystems are not equivalent in their capacities however. With the progressive uncoupling of system and lifeworld, the media, and thus subsytems, of the former come to dominate the latter. Habermas writes in this connection of the 'colonization' of the lifeworld. In a manner linked directly to the Weberian theme of rationalization and the Marxian theme of commodification, the lifeworld becomes colonized, 'that is increasingly state administered ("juridified") and commercialized. Possibilities for communicative action in the lifeworld become attenuated as social participation becomes hyper-rationalized in terms of immediate returns. Participants encounter each other as legal entities and as parties to contracts rather than as thinking and acting subjects' (Crook *et al.*, 1992: 28). System rationalization has outstripped the rationalization of the lifeworld: in other words, western rationalization has been 'selective'. The relations between system and lifeworld from the perspective of the former are summarized in Figure 1.1.

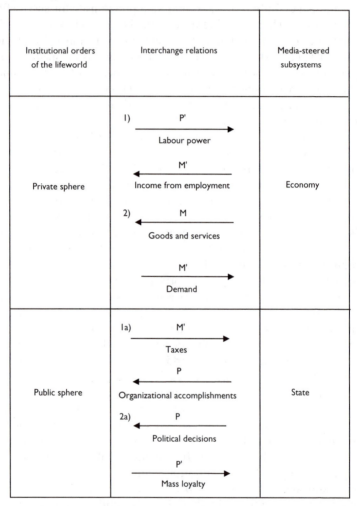

Figure 1.1   Relations between system and lifeworld from the perspective of the system

Source: Adapted from Habermas, 1987

Note: M = Money medium; P = Power medium

As indicated earlier, however, for all that Habermas agrees that western rationalization has proved selective in this sense, he distances himself from the 'iron cage' pessimism of Weber and others. He accuses Weber of treating the rationalization that has occurred in the Occident as inevitable when it was in fact contingent and selective. Weber, in short, is charged with conflating the *dynamic* and the *logic* of development. Habermas maintains that the logic of development allows for further rationalization of the lifeworld – that is, for an extension of the scope for communicative action and communicative rationality – and, it follows, for lifeworld 'decolonization', notably through a reconstitution of its public sphere. Currently the most likely, if as yet admittedly unlikely, agents of such a reconstitution, and of a reconstructed project of modernity, are the 'new', as opposed to the older class-based, social movements. Even Habermas sees little prospect of short-term gains.

Discourse ethics

Habermas' (1990a, 1993) discourse ethics represents an elaboration or deepening of his theory of communicative action; and as such it too remains at the formal or procedural level. At its core is a *principle of universalization*, which represents a 'socialization' of Kant's individualistic moral theory in line with objections penned initially by Hegel. This principle is intended to compel the 'universal exchange of roles' termed 'ideal role taking' or 'universal discourse' by Mead. Thus every valid norm has to fulfil the following condition: '*all* affected can accept the consequences and the side effects its *general* observance can be anticipated to have for the satisfaction of *everyone's* interests (and these consequences are preferred to those of known alternative possibilities for regulation)' (Habermas, 1990: 65; original emphasis).

The principle of universalization should not be confused with the *principle of discourse ethics*, which states that 'only those norms can claim to be valid that meet (or could meet) with the approval of all affected in their capacity *as participants in a practical discourse*' (Habermas, 1990: 66; original emphasis). While the principle of universalization concerns *moral* questions of 'justice' and 'solidarity', which admit of formal universal solution, the principle of discourse ethics concerns *ethical* questions of the 'good life', which can only be addressed in the context of substantive cultures, forms of life or individual projects.

Discourse ethics accords priority to moral questions of justice and solidarity. And justice and solidarity are necessarily related and of the essence of communicative action. Justice here refers to the 'subjective freedom of inalienable individuality'; and solidarity refers to the 'well-being of associated members of a community who intersubjectively share the same lifeworld' (Habermas, 1990: 200). Morality, according to Habermas (1990: 200), 'cannot protect the rights of the individual without also protecting the well-being of the community to which he belongs'. One of his expositors, Rehg, is worth quoting at length on this (see also Scambler, 1998):

> Contrary to Descartes, one arrives at rational conviction not in isolation but only in a public space, however such a certain solitude might be necessary as one moment in this process. We thus find justice linked – at its very basis in rational autonomy – with a real dependence on others' rational autonomy. For in as much as my conviction about moral obligation cannot come at the expense of yours, in disregard for your inviolable right to say no, it must submit itself to the testing of the deliberating community of all those affected. Precisely the effort to convince others of the justice of a normative expectation demands that I attend emphatically to its effects on others' welfare. Both the community whose cooperative structures are at stake in moral deliberation as well as the concrete others involved in such cooperation enter into the very constitutions of justice under the aegis of rational solidarity.
>
> (Rehg, 1994: 245)

Habermas' claims for his discourse ethics are restricted. As a moral theory, discourse ethics purports to 'ground the moral point of view', to clarify the 'universal core of moral intuitions' and to 'refute value scepticism'. What it cannot and does not aim to do is resolve substantive issues. 'By singling out a procedure of decision-making, it seeks to make room for those involved, who must then find answers on their own to the moral-practical issues that come at them, or are imposed on them, with objective historical force' (Habermas, 1990: 211).

The law, rights and deliberative democracy

In *Between Facts and Norms* (1996), and in several of the papers in *The Inclusion of the Other* (1998a), Habermas builds on his discourse ethics to shed further light on the law and democracy. His position has been neatly summarized by Cronin and De Greiff (1998: vii), who write: 'Extending his discourse theory of normative validity to the legal-political domain, he defends a proceduralist conception of deliberative democracy in which the burden of legitimating state power is borne by informal and legally institutionalized processes of political deliberation. Its guiding intuition is the radical democratic idea that the legitimacy of political authority can only be secured through broad popular participation in political deliberation and decision-making or, more succinctly, that there is an internal relation between the rule of law and popular sovereignty.'

One way of interpreting Habermas' analysis here is as an attempt to accommodate what is commendable in 'liberalism', focused predominantly on autonomy, on the one hand, and what is commendable in 'communitarianism', focused predominantly on legitimacy, on the other, while moving beyond that which is indefensible in each approach. Both classical liberalism and communitarianism assume that morality represents a higher domain of value in which basic legal and political principles must be grounded, the former stressing pre-politically grounded rights of individual liberty, and the latter values emergent in culturally trans-mitted religious, ethnic or national identities which form the inescapable background against which all questions of political justice must be answered. Against both approaches, Habermas argues that morality and law stand in a 'complementary relation': moreover, the core human rights enshrined in legal orders are essentially *legal*, not moral, rights.

Habermas contends that doing justice to the distinctive mode of legitimacy of positive legal orders requires consideration of just which basic rights free and equal citizens must confer on one another if they are to regulate their common life by means of posi-tive law. These rights fall into five categories. The first triad constitutes the fundamental negative liberties: they are those membership rights and due-process rights that together guarantee private autonomy. The fourth are rights of political participation that guarantee public autonomy. And the fifth are social-welfare rights, necessary in that the effective exercise of civil and political rights depends on certain social and material conditions (e.g. that citizens can meet basic material needs). The policing power of state authority is required to enforce and stabilize such a system of rights; and this introduces a new tension, namely, that between state power and legitimate law. Habermas insists that an account of public reason is vital, and that this must ultimately refer to democractic processes of opinion- and will-formation in the public sphere. In this way he seeks to link the informal discursive sources of democracy with the formal decision-making institutions necessary for the effective rule of law in complex societies. His argument is that it is in fact the constitu-tional state that represents the crucial network of legal institutions and mechanisms that governs the conversion of citizens' commu-nicative power into legitimate administrative activity. Law, he writes, 'represents ... the medium for transforming communicative power into administrative power' (Habermas, 1996: 159; see Scambler, 1998a).

For Habermas, then, the legitimacy of legal norms is a function of those formal properties of procedures of political deliberation and decision making that support the presumption that their outcomes are rational. What criteria would the requisite institutions have to meet? Habermas writes of the needs, first, for a public sphere of open political discussion, characterized by inputs of expert knowledge and by ready access to print and electronic media, and institutionally underwritten by the voluntary associations of civil society. This public sphere would be complemented, second, by a legally regulated government sphere consisting of legislative, judi-cial and administrative branches. While this model is contiguous with the arrangements of most modern constitutional democracies, Habermas' rationale, in terms of the legitimating function of public reason, is original. Cronin and De Greiff (1998: xvii) refer to his model as involving the *circulation of power*: 'on the input side, influ-ence generated in the public sphere is transformed through the democratic procedures of elections and parliamentary opinion- and will-formation into communicative power; which in turn is trans-formed through the legal programmes and policies of parliamentary bodies into administrative power; at the output end, administrative programmes create the necessary conditions for the existence of civil society and its voluntary associations, and hence of a vibrant political public sphere'.

Mention might finally be made of Habermas' (1998a) linkage of these arguments in his most recent writings with the future of the nation-state in an era of globalization. He argues that the kind of republicanism he favours must be preserved at the supranational level if it is to be preserved at all. This is so because individual nation-states now suffer from three relevant weaknesses: first, they no longer have the resources to tackle risks on a global scale, including ecological crises, economic inequalities, the arms trade and international crime; second, they are becoming relatively help-less in the face of the globalization or de-nationalization of the economy; and third, they now experience an inherent tension between nationalism and republicanism which makes them less than reliable guarantors of human rights, as opposed to those rights that accrue to citizens of particular states. It hardly needs appending that, for all his democratic cosmopolitan orientation, Habermas remains highly critical of extant supranational bodies like the United Nations and the European Parliament (see Rosenfeld and Arato, 1998).

Arguments, suggestions and pointers

Many of Habermas' contributions, and even of his public interven-tions, occur at the interface of philosophy and sociology. Many too embody a recognition that problems once regarded as (purely) philosophical can no longer be solved in the absence of a deep and informed sense of society (in some respects an 'Hegelianization' of Kant, as well as an aspect of what Kilminster (1998) presents as a more recent 'sociological revolution'). While it might be thought that much of this work is, strictly speaking, superfluous to soci-ology's needs, there are two obvious senses in which this is questionable. First, at a time when the very pursuit of a 'modernist' sociology is under attack, Habermas' reconstruction of the Enlightenment or 'modernist' project through his theory of commu-nicative action might be held to be an opportune and signal piece of analysis. Second, this same analysis, arising out of unambiguously acknowledged deficiencies in the previously unreconstructed Enlightenment project, pulls the rug from beneath the feet of many species of 'postmodernist', exposing their members as muddled relativists and neo-conservative apologists for the status quo (Habermas, 1987a, 1989a).

Worthy of reflection too is the import of what might be termed the *counterfactual character* of crucial aspects of Habermas' work, early and late. It is the counterfactual suggestiveness of the ideal speech situation (in its early and late formulations), for example, which provides critical edge, affording a standard against which to evaluate strategic action in all its guises and disguises. No less counterfactually suggestive is the formal or procedural presentation of 'free-floating public communication' as of the essence of the public sphere of the lifeworld, promising a means for the exposure of anti-democratic practice and other forms of system colonization of the lifeworld in high modernity.

The conceptual framework elaborated most comprehensively in *Theory of Communicative Action*, consisting of a progressively uncoupled system and lifeworld, replete with their respective – if asymmetrical – subsystems and steering media, and explicitly intended by Habermas to have empirical as well as methodological potency, has a fulsome and largely untapped potential to shape and inform theories of the changing character of modernity and of its social institutions, including those around health and illness. The whole issue of the delineation, enactment and monitoring of criteria of appropriateness in relation to the balance between system and lifeworld inputs to health and healing is a stark case in point.

More substantively yet, Habermas' more straightforwardly socio-logical writings on the bourgeois public sphere and, in its most Marxist vein, on crises of legitimation in advanced capitalist societies, both updated and revised by him since their initial publication, have spawned immense literatures. Both hold promise for analysis of health and health care. Recent accounts of civil society and the public sphere, for example, have focused attention increasingly on the salience of (new) social movements forming at the junctures of system and lifeworld and geared to the defence and decolonization of the latter. Appraisals of the seriousness of the threats of crises of legitimation that face governments increasingly (having to) promise their electorates more than they are able to deliver are particularly pertinent to considerations of health care and other welfare spending 'cuts' into the early years of the twenty-first century.

The chapters that follow cover a broad range of areas and topics in the health arena for which Habermas' work has relevance. Gareth Williams and Jennie Popay draw on their own study to reflect on the nature of lay health knowledge. They suggest that there is a – often neglected or overlooked – 'ferment of critical thinking' in the life-world, for the most part contained within its private sphere, which betrays 'an understanding of the complex interplay of biography, history, locality, and the broader social divisions of class and gender'. They employ a Habermasian perspective to question the simple distinctions between expert and non-expert in the field of public health and commend further explorations of the 'rationalities of everyday life'. Nicky Britten and I deploy the system–lifeworld distinction to contextualize both macro and micro approaches to doctor–patient interaction. Focusing on increasingly topical issues of trust, we maintain that Habermas' notions of selective rationalization and lifeworld colonization have direct relevance to understanding the doctor–patient relationship. Specifically, phenomena like clientalism and consumerism can be shown to routinely distort doctor–patient interaction despite both parties acting in good faith and with reciprocal satisfaction.

Ian Rees Jones uses Habermas' theory of communicative action as a framework for a critical analysis of decision making in health care. With particular reference to the key but 'ambivalent' role of public health practitioners as decision makers and mediators, he shows how and why their engagement requires to be understood as political rather than technical. In the following chapter on class, power and health inequalities, I attempt to make plausible what I term the 'greedy bastards hypothesis' (or GBH), which asserts that health inequalities in Britain can reasonably be understood as indirect (and largely unintended) consequences of the ever-adaptive behaviours of members of the power elite and capitalist-executive. The GBH makes genuinely sociological notions of class and power central to explaining contemporary health inequalities. David Kelleher then considers the role and potential of new social movements in the domain of health, arguing that 'some' self-help groups, insofar as they provide their members with 'the opportunity to construct personal and joint narratives', and then allow them to relate and question accounts, can be seen as engaged in resisting lifeworld colonization.

Paul Higgs and Ian Rees Jones demonstrate that 'the struggle between technocratic and popular appoaches to the issue of rationing health care is ultimately a political conflict'. They contend that current debates about rationing conceal deep contradictions in the modern world, stressing the salience of the concept of 'class-based ideology' for attempts to understand these contradictions. Ian Rees Jones follows this by asking whether the studies of Habermas and Foucault are opposed or complementary. Through a discussion of medicalization, globalization, governmentality and surveillance, he reaches the conclusion that a Habermasian framework has some advantages over a Foucauldian framework because it allows for a critical perspective, avoids postmodern traps of conservatism and nihilism and has the greater democratic reach. And in the final chapter Leslie Martin and I dwell on the notions of civil society, the public sphere and deliberative democracy, making a case that there are logical and moral ties between these and the pursuit of a critical sociology. The significance and possibility of alliances between critical sociologists and new social movement and other lifeworld activists towards the institutionalization of avenues of deliberative democracy is discussed.

References

Austin, J. (1962) *How To Do Things With Words*. Oxford: Oxford University Press.
Beetham, D. (1991) *The Legitimation of Power*. London: Macmillan.
Beilharz, P. (1995) 'Critical theory – Jürgen Habermas'. In Roberts, D. (ed.) *Reconstructing Theory: Gadamer, Habermas, Luhman*. Melbourne: Melbourne University Press.
Best, S. and Kellner, D. (1991) *Postmodern Theory: Critical Interrogations*. London: Macmillan.
Braaten, J. (1991) *Habermas' Critical Theory of Society*. New York: State University of New York Press.
Brand, A. (1990) *The Force of Reason: An Introduction to Habermas' 'Theory of Communicative Action'*. London: Allen & Unwin.
Calhoun, C. ed.(1992) *Habermas and the Public Sphere*. Cambridge, MA: MIT Press.
Cronin, C. and De Greiff, P. (1998) 'Introduction'. In Habermas, J., *The Inclusion of the Other: Studies in Political Theory*. Cambridge: Polity Press.
Crook, S., Paluski, J. and Waters, M. (1992) *Postmodernization: Changes in Advanced Society*. London: Sage.
Giddens, A. (1985) 'Jürgen Habermas'. In Skinner, Q. (ed.) *The Return of Grand Theory in the Human Sciences*. Cambridge: Cambridge University Press.
Habermas, J. (1976) *Legitimation Crisis*. London: Heinemann.
—— (1981) 'Modernity versus postmodernity'. *New German Critique*, 22: 3–11.
—— (1984) *The Theory of Communicative Action, Volume One: Reason and the Rationalization of Society*. London: Heinemann.
—— (1986) *Theory and Practice*. Cambridge: Polity Press.
—— (1986a) *Towards a Rational Society*. Cambridge: Polity Press.

—— (1986b) *Knowledge and Human Interests*. Cambridge: Polity Press.
—— (1987) *The Theory of Communicative Action, Volume Two: Lifeworld and System: A Critique of Functionalist Reason*. Cambridge: Polity Press.
—— (1987a) *The Philosophical Discourse of Modernity*. Cambridge: Polity Press.
—— (1989) *The Structural Transformation of the Public Sphere: an Inquiry into a Category of Bourgeois Society*. Cambridge: Polity Press.
—— (1989a) *The New Conservatism*. Cambridge: Polity Press.
—— (1990) *On the Logic of the Social Sciences*. Cambridge: Polity Press.
—— (1990a) *Moral Consciousness and Communicative Action*. Cambridge: Polity Press.
—— (1991) *Communication and the Evolution of Society*. Cambridge: Polity Press.
—— (1992) 'Further reflections on the public sphere'. In Calhoun, C. (ed.) *Habermas and the Public Sphere*. Cambridge, MA: MIT Press.
—— (1993) *Justification and Application: Remarks on Discourse Ethics*. Cambridge: Polity Press.
—— (1996) *Between Facts and Norms: Contributions to a Discourse Theory of Law and Democracy*. Cambridge: Polity Press.
—— (1998) *On the Pragmatics of Communication*. Cambridge: Polity Press.
—— (1998a) *The Inclusion of the Other: Studies in Political Theory*. Cambridge: Polity Press.
Holub, R. (1991) *Jürgen Habermas: Critic in the Public Sphere*. London: Routledge.
Horkheimer, M. and Adorno, T. (1982) *Dialectic of Enlightenment*. New York: Continuum.
Kant, I. (1970) 'An answer to the question "What is Enlightenment?"'. In Reiss, H. (ed.) *Kant's Political Writings*. Cambridge: Cambridge University Press.
Kilminster, R. (1998) *The Sociological Revolution*. London: Routledge.
Lawrence, P. (1989) 'The state and legitimation: the work of Jürgen Habermas'. In Duncan, G. (ed.) *Democracy and the Capitalist State*. Cambridge: Cambridge University Press.
McCarthy, T. (1978) *The Critical Theory of Jürgen Habermas*. Cambridge: Polity Press.
Outhwaite, W. (1996) 'Introduction'. In Outhwaite, W. (ed.) *The Habermas Reader*. Cambridge: Polity Press.
—— (1996a) *Habermas: A Critical Introduction*. Cambridge: Polity Press.
Ray, L. (1993) *Rethinking Critical Theory: Emancipation in the Age of Global Social Movements*. London: Sage.
Rehg, W. (1994) *Insight and Solidarity: The Discourse Ethics of Jürgen Habermas*. Berkeley: University of California Press.
Rockmore, T. (1989) *Habermas on Historical Materialism*. Bloomington and Indianapolis: Indiana University Press.

Rosenfeld, M. and Arato, A. (eds) (1998) *Habermas on Law and Democracy: Critical Exchanges*. Berkeley: University of California Press.

Scambler, G. (1987) 'Habermas and the power of medical expertise'. In Scambler, G. (ed.) *Sociological Theory and Medical Sociology*. London: Tavistock.

—— (1996) 'The "project of modernity" and the parameters for a critical sociology: an argument with illustrations from medical sociology'. *Sociology*, 30: 567–81.

—— (1998) 'Medical sociology and modernity: reflections on the public sphere and the roles of intellectuals and social critics'. In Scambler, G. and Higgs, P. (eds) *Modernity, Medicine and Health: Medical Sociology Towards 2000*. London: Routledge.

—— (1998a) 'Theorizing modernity: Luhmann, Habermas, Elias and new perspectives on health and healing'. *Critical Public Health*, 8: 237–44.

Schmidt, J. (1982) 'Jürgen Habermas and the difficulties of Enlightenment'. *Social Research*, 49.

Scott, J. (1995) *Sociological Theory: Contemporary Debates*. Aldershot: Edward Elgar Publishing Company.

Sitton, J. (1996) *Recent Marxian Theory: Class Formation and Social Conflict in Contemporary Capitalism*. New York: State University of New York Press.

Thompson, J. (1984) 'Rationality and social rationalization: an assessment of Habermas' theory of communicative action'. In Thompson, J. (ed.) *Studies in the Theory of Ideology*. Cambridge: Polity Press.

Chapter 2

Lay health knowledge and the concept of the lifeworld

Gareth Williams and Jennie Popay

Introduction

The exploration of lay perspectives on health and illness now has a long, convoluted and multidisciplinary history, but its place within medical sociology can be understood to reflect some of sociology's more ubiquitous historically embedded ideological concerns.

To a greater degree than is the case in the other social sciences, within sociology there has been a tradition of partisan research and theorizing in which being on the side of the 'wretched of the earth' was a necessary prelude to the production of any kind of worthwhile sociology. This is characteristically, although not necessarily, taken to entail some kind of commitment to left-wing, left-leaning, or subversive political ideology, a profound mistrust of the holders of political and economic power, and a belief that traditional positivistic methods of research are both epistemologically too blunt, and ethically too tainted by their association with the institutions of the establishment. Doing life histories or participant observation is seen as a way of getting inside the lives of individuals and groups who are outside the power structures, with a view to telling it like it is: a sociological version of history from below (Thompson, 1963).

The 1960s and 1970s saw the appearance of a proliferation of methodological approaches that were more like anthropology or campaigning journalism – the old journalism of Henry Mayhew (Thompson and Yeo, 1971, 1973) or the 'new journalism' of Tom Wolfe – than the conventional sociology undertaken by a 'dry character with an insatiable lust for statistics' (Berger, 1979: 11). But these were not only questions of 'method' in the narrow sense. They were challenges to the fundamental orientation of sociology and the social sciences to the power structures in which such activities were embedded. Being a critical sociologist meant positioning oneself in a particularly partisan way in relation to the task of researching and writing about expressions of power. Medical sociology's particular version of this – a version that persuaded many that the discipline was not just a question of helping doctors do their jobs better – was a radical approach which took the side of the patients against the doctors as agents of social control (Zola, 1972; Illich, 1975) or – in some versions – an arm of the capitalist state (Navarro, 1978).

The most recent discrediting of Marxism, communism and even socialism by events in Eastern Europe and elsewhere has provided the opportunity for a whole range of marketeers, spin doctors and philosophers of the end of history to rise gloriously on the crest of a resurgent wave of global capitalism. Faced with the argument and the apparent reality that global capitalism is all there is – and you had better get used to it even if you are not in a position to enjoy it – it has become increasingly difficult to find genuinely oppositional alternative standpoints, apart from being 'anti-capitalist' in the rather general and diffuse, if highly organized, manner of recent socio-environmental movements. Those ways of thinking critically which were so central to intellectual opposition in British universities, political parties and social movements up to the middle of the 1980s; those thinkers who were so much part of the personal and professional history of those who came to the social sciences during the late 1960s and after; and those assumptions about established and alternative ways of being and doing with which activists oriented themselves to personal and public life, have become increasingly uncertain and unreliable guides.

There were, of course, people who never did warm to what they saw as left-wing posturing; and there were those who underwent a kind of Pauline conversion to the benefits of markets and the illusions of socialism with almost unseemly haste (Selborne, 1985). All this had its effects too within the circumscribed boundaries of medical sociology. Some of those arguments *against* the medical profession, those unchallengeable criticisms of bureaucracy, those sure-fire positions of opposition against known enemies – corruptly powerful hospital consultants, avaricious drug companies, inept general practitioners and indifferent nurses – are no longer so easily bought. On the other hand, part of the ideological reconstruction of capitalism has included a rhetoric of consumerism, which, paradoxically, provides support (in some versions) for the patient against what are seen as the market-perverting special interests of professional power.

Some of this breaking up of ritual position-taking and ideological posturing is no doubt a welcome sign of progress and maturity; a movement away from entrenched positions and name-calling across perceived ideological divides. But the loss of such coordinates also produces that sense of ambivalence which makes us unable properly to understand what is going on and to decide what course of action to take (Bauman, 1991). Within the study of health and illness, as in other fields, some have embraced the new indeterminacy with excitement, finding themselves able to develop new perspectives on bodies, minds and human relationships that are, to coin a phrase, 'beyond left and right' (Giddens, 1994; Williams, S. *et al.*, 2000); a third way which can encompass a truly startling array of ideologies, beliefs and arguments. Others have absorbed the arguments of Foucault, Lyotard and other postmodern and post-structuralist thinkers. Their nuanced approach to power and freedom has facilitated novel ways of thinking about relationships between bodies, individuals and a range of knowledges and discourses which in one way or another construct illness realities and relationships between lay and professional groups.

What is characteristic of much of this work is its willingness to explore cultures, knowledges, and discourses as realities *sui generis*, without reference to political economy or history. Much of this work has taken to heart the end of history, the death of Marxism and the universalization of global markets, and has either abandoned any interest in 'liberation sociology' or has attempted to unfold its radicalism within multiple, fragmented discursive realms. And yet alongside this new intellectual and political pluralism, with its rejection of the overarching narratives suggested by Marxism or feminism, there is a continuing recognition of the overwhelming impact of material and structural forces on the major causes of mortality, morbidity and general unhappiness in western society (Marmot and Wilkinson, 1999; Shaw *et al.*, 1999). In contrast to the situation during the 1980s and early 1990s, it is possible once again to say that risks are distributed by material forces – even if they are also 'socially constructed' – and this distribution is systematically unequal.

However, the material circumstances experienced by the insecure citizen will provide the material for the development of understanding rooted in personal experience. Between the 'abstracted empiricism' of epidemiologists and the 'Grand Theory' of sociologists lies a form of knowledge that is empirical without being empiricist and theoretical without being grandiose. This is the knowledge developed by lay people, and re-developed by social scientists through the knowledge lay people bring, to understand and act upon the conditions of risk in which they find themselves. This knowledge is critical (in the best traditions of the Frankfurt School), and it is most certainly reflexive in the sense of being 'subject to... revision in the light of changing circumstances' (Williams, S. and Calnan, 1996: 1612). There is also a growing confidence among lay publics about the 'expertise' they gain from their personal experience (Popay and Williams, 1994). This reflects, in part, a wider public scepticism about 'professional expertise' that will be an important context for researching the people's health in the future.

Habermas' concepts of 'system' and 'lifeworld'

Although Habermas himself remains one of the bridges to classical sociological traditions and one of the originators of contemporary social theory, even at the peak of his esteem and popularity it was never entirely easy to see how he related to the ordinary concerns of everyday life, or indeed everyday social sciences. He has remained resistant to simple incorporation into the conduct of empirical research. For all the difficulties of his archaeologies and genealogies, Foucault at least seemed to write very directly about prisons, hospitals and asylums in a way that informed the empirical research and policy analysis of people working in those specific areas. Habermas, in contrast, while being the author of many think-pieces about contemporary events, has written virtually nothing about the social institutions and processes – schools, benefit offices, health services – through which we experience the wider societal distribution of power, status and wealth. While according a measure of intellectual respect to Foucault, Habermas has been a staunch opponent to what he sees as the fripperies of postmodernist thinking (Habermas, 1987).

In the condition of ambivalence in which we find ourselves today, with Grand Narratives crumbling literally right, left and centre (and multiple screams, songs and short stories arising from the rubble), and with a growing obsession with evidence and the interface with policy and real-world decision making, it is even less easy to see what he can possibly say that will help us negotiate this 'runaway world'. Nonetheless, there have been those working within the highly empirical and applied world of modern medical sociology who have continued to insist on his relevance to the very practical problems of everyday life, including those of ill health, and the organization of activities for dealing with them (Crossley, 2000).

Any discussion of the relevance of Habermas, of course, needs some qualification. After all, his work from the late 1960s onwards contains many chapters and a large number of interesting footnotes, and not only to Plato. There is also a degree of interconnectedness of many of his main ideas over almost four decades which makes it difficult to excise something from the corpus in a way that is valid and fair. Nonetheless, it seems to us that in trying to think about the world of everyday life in Habermasian terms, theoretical progress will only be made if we approach Habermas less as acolytes and more as jobbing sociologists trying to make sense of some piece of the social world and the role of our empirical research in it.

For the purposes of the ensuing discussion, we are particularly interested in the way in which work we have undertaken over the last few years on lay knowledge can be seen to owe something, although neither consciously nor explicitly, to some of Habermas' preoccupations. His concern with the deformation of the public sphere under conditions of advanced capitalism, for example; his critique of the way in which political decisions are re-defined as technical prescriptions; his perspective on the dominance of technique over praxis; and his arguments about the colonization of the lifeworld – in both public and private spheres – by the powers of the state and the forces of capitalism; and the possibilities of resistance within both politics and civil society. Although discussed by Habermas himself at a level of high theoretical abstraction, it seems to us that his ideas have a powerful bearing on empirically researchable issues of the relationship between lay and expert knowledge.

The grammar of forms of life

As Scambler suggests (see Chapter 1), in drawing on Weberian perspectives on rationalization and the Marxian analyses of commodification and alienation, Habermas points to the way in which the possibilities of praxis within the lifeworld have been attenuated as social life and action becomes hyperrationalized in terms of immediate, instrumentally or contractually defined returns. However, as Scambler also indicates, in different shades of contrast to Weber's pessimism and Marx's revolutionary eschatology and, it might be added, many forms of postmodernism, Habermas recognizes the possibility of points of resistance to the rationalization and globalization of economic and political systems, not through class struggle or party political reform, but through new movements of opposition arising within civil society. If many western societies are now characterized by the progressive fragmentation of class structures and class consciousness' (see Edgell, 1993: 120), then, as Habermas argues:

> The utopian idea of a society based on social labour has lost its persuasive power ... because that utopia has lost its point of reference in reality: the power of abstract labour to create structure and give form to society.
>
> (1989: 53)

The welfare state which developed in response to the earlier deprivations of capitalism has itself become part of the problem, intervening through the inspection and control of the everyday lives of ordinary working-class people (Habermas, 1989). The welfare state that can be seen to some extent to have emerged from reformist class conflict now stands in an alienated relationship to the people whom it was supposed to serve. From this viewpoint the class conflict is not the primary shaping force within these new forms of conflict. Rather, as Habermas has argued, they '... concern the *grammar of forms of life*' and '... arise at the seam between system and lifeworld' (1981: 33, 36).

One aspect of the 'grammar of forms of life' to which Habermas refers are the changing relationships of knowledge and power between 'lay' populations or citizens and the professional, certified experts who have become a proliferating feature of late capitalism. Desire for scientific certainty coexists with the uneasy recognition that this is not possible. The British Government, dealing with the many implications of the crisis over beef, draws upon the rhetoric of scientific neutrality and the importance of 'evidence' as opposed to 'gossip' (*Guardian*, 1996). However, it is perfectly plain to the man and woman in the butcher's shop, the farm and the abattoir that professional experts 'disagree', and that the nature of such disagreement often goes beyond any simple accumulation of epidemiological or other factual evidence. Expert knowledge is essentially contested, and experts are increasingly seen as integral to the world of politics and power which makes public opinion more suspicious of the quality of their judgements.

In a world of epistemological uncertainty and 'competing rationalities' there is no universal map to guide us, only a number of alternative projections (Curry, 1996). Local knowledge – in the sense of knowledge that lay people obtain in the daily routine of their lives – is seen by some as a failed or flawed form of scientific knowledge, or as something other than knowledge altogether. However, stimulated by developments in anthropology, lay knowledge derived from the particular – the particular locality, biography and body – is increasingly recognized as very rich and directed at different ends. Local knowledge as *material* knowledge provides understanding which is 'emplaced' (Curry, 1996).

While this may raise for some the prospect of a postmodern maelstrom or mania of perspectivism, subjectivism and relativism, we would see it rather as an opportunity for the development of dialogue across areas of expertise, lay and professional, and for exploring – although not without conflict – the understanding developed within different discourses. As Habermas himself argued some years ago:

> Our only hope for the rationalization of the power structure lies in conditions that favour political power for thought developing through dialogue.
>
> (Habermas, 1971: 61)

The material basis of lay knowledge

The concept of lay knowledge embodies a concern with the subjective views of lay people. However, as we have employed it in our work, it refers to the way in which those views are shaped in response to particular events and experiences which undermine security and are shaped by the conditions or circumstances in which people live. It is concerned with 'the grammar of forms of life' as these are embedded or emplaced within the material conditions of everyday life. Lay knowledge is an expression of lifeworld concerns that seeks a public forum but is often excluded from wider recognition by the 'system' forces of state and economy.

In a study we conducted in Salford some years ago (Williams *et al.*, 1997), we were funded by the local health promotion department to find out about what people living in the inner city saw as the main risks to their health. The aim of the research was to enable people to talk widely about what it was like living in the area and to explore their perceptions of the health-related risks they faced within the context of their daily lives. The study showed that people are very aware of the health-related risks they face, but that although aware of the effects of behavioural factors, such as smoking, drugs, drinking, diet and exercise on their health status, they were unable to make sense of these without contextualizing them in structural or material terms. In some accounts a range of specific problems were identified.

Health problems associated with poor housing, for example, were a persistent feature of people's experience of life in the area. People living in high-rise accommodation stressed the practical and psychological difficulties of bringing up children in this environment – feeling depressed and isolated, being unable physically to get in and out of the area because of faulty lifts; trying to negotiate the area with prams and shopping. Some respondents had found it difficult to obtain any stable and secure accommodation in the first place, being subject to numerous moves around the locality over relatively short periods of time.

Unemployment, poverty, economic decline and the experience of crime were frequently mentioned as having severe and debilitating effects on people's health. Some residents of the area found it difficult to identify specific factors damaging their health, but feeling generally 'stressed' was central to their experience. As one respondent commented:

> I think the biggest health risk is mentally ... 'cause it's a lot of pressure and there's nothing really for you to do ... you're sort of segregated all of the time'. (123)

In the context of a political system that would claim high degrees of system integration, the use of the term 'segregation' by a middle-aged white man has a startling effect. Moreover, while it is common to use the term 'pressure' when someone has too much to do, here we see pressure linked with having nothing to do and being 'segregated' from things to do and from other people. Segregation sounds much stronger than 'social exclusion' (which was not yet being talked about when these data were collected) although they might amount to the same thing. The former term connects our understanding of this man's experience of the life-world to racism, apartheid and imprisonment, and shocks us out of liberal assumptions about the nature and limits of poverty in British society.

Some of the people interviewed presented a sophisticated understanding of the structuration of health-related risk and behaviour:

> ... there are reasons why people are smoking. If they don't have a smoke then they are going round the twist and ending up going to the doctor for their nerves ... or having a drink. I put it down to the environment ... you'll find that in areas where people are poor ... what happens to these people when they are going on the dole is that they are living on nothing until their giro arrives and they are so depressed that they are going straight to the pub when the giro arrives and living on nothing until the next one arrives ... then they are back to being depressed afterwards. (124)

There was a widespread perception among the people interviewed in this study that many aspects of the local 'environment' had a substantial negative impact on the health experience of people living in this inner city area. This 'environment' was sometimes defined in terms of the absence of material amenities, for example, employment prospects, adequate incomes, decent housing, recreational facilities, parks, playgrounds and daycare for children. On other occasions it was defined in terms of the presence of phenomena that were detrimental to health: crime, traffic accidents, chemical pollution, discarded syringes, drugs, physical drabness and decay, and violence and disorder among the local population. And within the accounts people theorized the relationship between what was present and what was absent.

Professional 'experts' and local people may differ over their definition of the environment and its relationship to the experience of ill health. This was, as we have argued, evident in this study. The respondents emphasized structural problems in relation to their conception of the environment rather than focusing on personal risk-taking behaviour such as drinking, smoking, diet, exercise. Where they were mentioned, individual 'risky' behaviours were frequently explained by reference to 'trying to cope' with some aspect of daily life. One young woman explained:

> Well, I do reach for a ciggy when the baby gets out of control
> and goes running off. And I've seen my friends lighting up
> when they get a big bill or something like that. (125)

While another respondent vividly argued:

> [S]moking, and drinking and drug taking. I put it down to one
> thing ... until money is spent on these areas ... there doesn't
> seem much point in trying to stop people smoking and what
> else. As long as the environment is going down the pan people
> will go down with it. (125)

In an important sense the people interviewed were 'going down together': for among this small sample of people there was to a considerable degree a shared understanding of the problems they faced in their everyday lives; of the harm that it could and was doing to their health and that of their children and neighbours; and of their lack of power to change things. A sense of powerlessness and the burden of simply coping with the social and material difficulties they faced in this locality were starkly evident in many accounts. Although there was a clear sense of the shared nature of the material conditions in which people found themselves, a sense of what might collectively be done was less evident, and professionals, not surprisingly, often did little to support anything other than an individualized, professional response.

Lay and expert knowledge

Health professionals have long recognized that lay people have opinions about the causes of ill health experienced by themselves or others. However, too often these opinions are construed as interesting but in some ways misguided 'ways of knowing' about health and illness. Even within the social sciences, where much of the research into lay beliefs about health and illness has been undertaken, these beliefs are rarely presented as enhancing understanding about explanations for ill health. Typically, they may be studied in their own right as cultural products or considered important to the development of more effective health promotion policies – where they inform our understanding of the place of health and illness within the social and cultural orders of everyday life (Blaxter, 1983; Cornwell, 1984; Davison et al., 1991).

Social research has explored the types of explanations for poor health offered by lay people. As several studies have demonstrated, there is a tendency for those living in the poorest material conditions and, potentially therefore experiencing the poorest health, to be more likely than relatively advantaged groups to blame poor health on individual behaviour. This is a complex issue, linked in part to the research methods used, the nature of the questions asked of respondents, and the relationship between health and morality within the western world (Blaxter, 1990, 1993; Pill and Stott, 1985).

To a large extent this body of social science research denies lay knowledge a place at the aetiological table. Lay explanations are the object of research seeking to understand why people put forward different types of explanations rather than research to inform understanding about the causes of ill health. Additionally, as Blaxter (2000) points out, there have been few systematic attempts to link together epidemiological work on social inequalities in health and research into biographical lay perspectives on health and illness. This is curious because these approaches to research clearly have much to offer each other in enhancing the degree of generalizability and validity of findings from such studies, and in answering questions that one or the other leaves in suspension. There is good and growing evidence that professionals involved in public health research – whatever their discipline – ignore the aetiological insights of lay experts at their peril.

Brown and colleagues, in the USA, have highlighted the role of lay knowledge in understanding the causes of ill health in their studies of community responses to environmental problems (Brown, 1992). They have documented situations where lay people have identified a relationship between the experience of health problems in a local community and exposure to toxic wastes. In seeking to 'prove' their case these communities may have used traditional epidemiological methods, but the initial knowledge is experiential. Similar situations concerned with toxic waste have been documented in Britain (Williams and Popay, 1994).

Lay theories of causality are evident in other fields of public health. For example, local communities have attempted to highlight the relationship between the health problems they experience and exposure to pollution from nuclear installation and chemical processing plants, to damp or structurally unsafe housing, to industrial pollution, high traffic densities and open-cast mining (for example, Platt *et al.*, 1989; Phillimore and Moffatt, 1994; Rice and Roberts, 1994; Beynon *et al.*, 2000). Workers have frequently been the first to identify causal relationships between their working environment and patterns of disease, and the trade union movement has a long history of activism around health and safety issues (Frumkin and Kantrowitz, 1987; Watterson, 1993; Bloor, 1999). Similarly, the wives of victims of asbestosis are reported as complaining to coroners' courts that the deaths were due to exposure to something at work, long before modern science studied the problem (Roberts, 1994).

These early warnings are often ignored or discounted by scientists. In many instances the relationships at the centre of these examples of 'popular epidemiology' remain contested by professional scientific experts, or denied. In the case of the Camelford incident in Britain, where aluminium sulphate was accidentally tipped into a local water supply, for example, two 'expert' reports have concluded that the physical problems reported by local people were associated with 'all the worry and concern' and that 'the psychological harm could last a long time for some people' (Department of Health, 1991). Similarly, the research on the relationship between damp and childhood illnesses (Platt *et al.*, 1989) challenged the professional view that parental smoking was the major risk factor, highlighting a dose–response relationship between the prevalence of respiratory illness in children and exposure to damp in the home.

There is a common and pervasive assumption that the views of lay people or local residents will automatically and uncritically 'exaggerate' a problem, and a recognition of this among local people may well deflect them from confronting a 'scientific' issue head on (Beynon *et al.*, 2000). Professional experts may stress the methodological difficulties of 'proving' the relationship. For example, at a public meeting called to discuss the relationship between urban pollution and childhood asthma in the Docklands area of London, the local Director of Public Health warned that it would be difficult and costly to prove the effects of pollution on health (*Guardian*, 1991). Long periods of time may pass during which no action will be taken or long legal battles may be waged. Meanwhile exposure continues, lay experts are ignored and lives are unnecessarily lost or damaged.

We have noted many reasons why the knowledge lay experts bring with them is ignored or discounted in research into the causes of contemporary health problems. A final factor worthy of mention is the prominent role of women as informal guardians of public health. Women's role in this regard has been widely documented within the family, within the informal care sector and within the world of paid health work (Graham, 1993). The fact that it is women who are often at the heart of lay action for health further re-enforces the tendency for professional scientists to discount lay knowledge. As Brown and Ferguson argue, the validity of the knowledge of women involved in toxic waste activism

> ... is contested by scientific experts and professionals, whose cultural beliefs about women and science lead them to refuse to accept the women activists' claims about the consequences of toxic waste.
>
> (Brown and Ferguson, 1995)

It would be an oversimplification to refer to lay knowledge and expert knowledge as if they were distinct, separable bodies of understanding. Experts are also lay people whose knowledge is framed by their experiences, and lay knowledge contains elements of expertise, accredited or otherwise. However, in so far as lay knowledge emerges from alienation, dissent and, sometimes, organized movements of opposition between system and lifeworld, it provides new ways of thinking about problems whose definition is conventionally dominated by professional experts.

The contested nature of knowledge

For the most part, scientists working within fields dominated by the biomedical perspective are not preoccupied by their epistemological assumptions, and it is in the nature of 'normal science' that this should be so. They appear to be entirely pragmatic and, therefore, reasonable and fair – but only within limits. As a recent editorial in a leading medical journal puts it:

> Research on the health of populations is still dominated by experimental designs based on simplistic notions of causality that try to remove the variation and complexity of real-life health and disease processes.
>
> (*Lancet*, 1994: 429)

Science imposes definite constraints, in normal times, upon what methods scientists can use, what procedures they can adopt, how, when and where results are to be published. In other words there are definite assumptions, held by powerful people, about what is considered properly scientific. Scientists might claim that they are only involved in making sure that what attempts to pass itself off as science is not dictated by the sectional interests of particular scientists. However, as Habermas suggested over twenty years ago:

> Because science must secure the objectivity of its statements against the pressure and seduction of particular interests, it deludes itself about the fundamental interests to which it owes not only its impetus but the *conditions of possible objectivity* themselves.
>
> (1978: 311; original emphasis)

Habermas' critique of western science is essentially a critique of ideology. That is, it is critical of the 'scientism' of science which attempts to give the impression that science, and in particular those forms of science which can be conducted in controlled settings, is the only form of activity through which knowledge of the world can be developed. Not only are other kinds of beliefs, perspectives, points of view and ideas not science: they are poor knowledge.

Such a limited and technocratic definition of testable knowledge militates against the development of understanding in areas which are less amenable to control among people whose ideas cannot easily be formulated as conventional hypothetico-deductive hypotheses. While the influence of Popper (1972) has fostered deductive thinking within epidemiology and public health, it has simultaneously inhibited the methodological pluralism and critical openness which research requires to deal with the problems confronting public health today (Pearce and Crawford-Brown, 1989; Burrage, 1987). It is this kind of epistemological hegemony against which 'critical theory' reacted (Adorno *et al.*, 1976), seeing it as something which had implications beyond science itself. It not only discounted certain forms of knowledge from entering scientific discussion, it also disempowered groups of people working outside the dominant paradigm from making any contribution to debate over the policies which science could inform (Habermas, 1971).

The theoretical critique of the positivist demarcation of science from non-science has provided the foundation for a much stronger critique of the 'rationality' of science from within the social sciences. Different sciences and approaches to science have, to use Habermas' term, different 'knowledge-guiding interests' (Habermas, 1978). These knowledge-guiding interests provide the conditions of possible objectivity within the framework of particular disciplines and forms of scientific and scholarly research. Successful science, far from conforming to Merton's norms of universality, communality, scepticism and disinterestedness (Merton, 1973), is based on the persistent lobbying of governmental representatives and the mobilization of a variety of other social groups in support of the scientists' interests, social groups which include 'the public'. As a commentary on science policy in the USA concluded: 'Science does not have an inherent entitlement to funding but it should try harder to get the public on its side' (*Lancet*, 1994a: 368).

One cannot study the context of science out of relation to its content, or vice versa. Following a Latourian line, Bartley has argued:

> If we separate the inside and outside of science ... we will be unable to understand the processes involved. Science must be studied in the context of the issue communities in which it is embedded.
>
> (Bartley, 1990: 383)

Work on the philosophy and sociology of science and the contested nature of knowledge does not provide an immediate justification for looking at lay knowledge as an important component of public health research. However, such a perspective helps to illuminate the dynamics of movements of opposition demanding not only a say in decisions on the siting of toxic industries and material (such as nuclear dumps), for example, but also a voice in the discussion over the evidence and theories for and against the likely health effects of such decisions. Moreover, the notion that science is part of an issue community in the same way as are more overtly partisan groupings is an important advance on the belief that science is in some sense privileged and untainted by worldly concerns.

Conclusion: lay knowledge and the politics of the lifeworld

We argue that there is no sure foundation to our knowledge, and that knowledge is not determined by the painstaking accumulation of empirical information (Bryant, 1995). These post-positivist assumptions inform our central contention that individuals are human agents who are knowledgeable about their society and capable of acting in it (Giddens, 1979, 1990). Bearing in mind the multiple meanings of 'critical' and 'critique' within critical theory, the research on lay knowledge in specific and identifiable social and material contexts serves as an illustration of the ferment of critical thinking within the lifeworld that is confined for the most part to private contexts, but threatens to emerge, and sometimes succeeds in emerging, into the public sphere. As Habermas argues:

> It is only under pressure of approaching problems that relevant components of such background knowledge are torn out of their unquestioned familiarity and brought to consciousness as something in need of being ascertained. It takes an earthquake to make us aware that we had regarded the ground on which we stand everyday as unshakable.
>
> (Habermas, 1984: 400–1)

For some people, of course, there are little earthquakes taking place every day, emerging out of their conditions of poverty, exclusion and even segregation. The work we have discussed here shows a range of ways in which lay knowledge embodies resistance to the colonization of the lifeworld by either the state or market forces. In the case of our own study, we can see how even in essentially personal accounts of the sort we collected the 'political' dimensions of population health, the complex and sophisticated knowledge that local people hold, and the embeddedness of behaviour in social relationships and material circumstances are clearly displayed.

These accounts show us not just that individuals experience society in interesting ways, but that the knowledge people have of the impact of social forces upon them contains an understanding of the complex interplay of biography, history, locality and the broader social divisions of class and gender. Contrary to what some professional experts may believe (see Trichopoulos, 1996), critical thinking is alive and well among 'the general public', whether or not they have heard of Popper's falsification criterion. The perspectives developed by Habermas provide a reason for collapsing simple distinctions of expert and non-expert in the field of public health. His theoretical construction of the relationship between system and lifeworld justifies the exploration of rationalities in everyday life, and alerts us to the material and historical grounding of subjectivity out of which deliberative democracy in the public health field can be developed.

References

Adorno, T., Albert, H., Dahrendorf, R., Habermas, J., Pilot, H. and Popper, K.R. (1976) *The Positivist Dispute in German Sociology*. London: Heinemann

Bartley, M. (1990) 'Do we need a strong programme in medical sociology?' *Sociology of Health and Illness*, 12: 371–90.

Bauman, Z. (1991) *Modernity and Ambivalence*. Cambridge: Polity Press.

Berger, P. (1979) *Facing Up to Modernity*. Harmondsworth: Penguin.

Beynon, H., Cox, A. and Hudson, R. (2000) *Digging Up Trouble: The Environmental Protest and Open-Cast Coal Mining*. London: Rivers Oram Press.

Blaxter, M. (1983) 'The causes of disease: women talking'. *Social Science and Medicine*, 17: 59–69.

—— (1990) *Health and Lifestyles*. London: Routledge.

—— (1993) 'Why do the victims blame themselves?' In Radley, A. (ed.) *Worlds of Illness: Biographical and Cultural Perspectives on Health and Disease*. London: Routledge.

—— (2000) 'Class, time and biography'. In Williams, S., Gabe, J. and Calnan, M. (eds) *Health, Medicine and Society: Key Theories, Future Agendas*. London: Routledge.

Bloor, M. (1999) 'The South Wales Miners Federation, miners' lung and the instrumental use of expertise, 1900–1950'. *Social Studies of Science*, 29: 1–16.

Brown, P. (1992) 'Popular epidemiology and toxic waste contamination'. *Journal of Health and Social Behaviour*, 33: 267–81.

Brown, P. and Ferguson, F. (1992) 'Making a big stink: women's work, women's relationships and toxic waste activism'. Paper presented to the Annual Meeting of the American Sociological Association, Pittsburgh, Pennsylvania.

Bryant, C.G.A. (1995) *Practical Sociology: Post-Empiricism and the Reconstruction of Theory and Application*. Cambridge: Polity Press.

Burrage, H. (1987) 'Epidemiology and community health: a strained connection?' *Social Science and Medicine*, 25: 895–903.

Cornwell, J. (1984) *Hard Earned Lives: Accounts of Health and Illness from East London.* London: Tavistock Publications.

Crossley, N. (2000) 'Emotions, psychiatry and social order: a Habermasian approach'. In Williams, S., Gabe, J. and Calnan, M. (eds) *Health, Medicine and Society: Key Theories, Future Agendas.* London: Routledge.

Curry, H. (1996) 'Space and place in geographic decision-making'. In *Technical Expertise and Public Decisions*, Conference Proceedings. Princeton, NJ: Princeton University, pp. 311–18.

Davison, C., Davey-Smith, G. and Frankel, S. (1991) 'Lay epidemiology and the prevention paradox: the implications of coronary candidacy for health education'. *Sociology of Health and Illness*, 13, 1: 1–19.

Department of Health (1991) *Water Pollution at Lowermoor, North Cornwall: Second Report of the Lowermoor Incident Health Advisory Group* (Chair: Dame Barbara Clayton). London: HMSO.

Edgell, S. (1993) *Class.* London: Routledge.

Frumkin, H. and Kantrowitz, W. (1987) 'Cancer clusters in the work place: an approach to investigation'. *Journal of Occupational Medicine*, 29: 949–52.

Giddens, A. (1979) *Central Problems in Social Theory: Action, Structure and Contradiction in Social Analysis.* London: Macmillan.

—— (1990) *The Consequences of Modernity.* Cambridge: Polity Press.

—— (1994) *Beyond Left and Right: The Future of Radical Politics.* Cambridge: Polity Press.

Graham, H. (1993) *Hardship and Health in Women's Lives.* Brighton: Harvester/Wheatsheaf.

Guardian (1991) 'Dusting down to fight in Docklands'.11 September, p. 21.

——(1996) 'Hiding behind experts' (editorial). 26 March.

Habermas, J. (1971) *Toward a Rational Society.* London: Heinemann.

—— (1978) *Knowledge and Human Interests* (second edition). London: Heinemann.

—— (1981) 'New social movements'. *Telos*, 49: 33–7.

—— (1984) *The Theory of Communicative Action, Volume One: Reason and the Rationalization of Society.* Boston: Beacon Press.

—— (1987) *The Theory of Communicative Action, Volume Two: Lifeworld and System: A Critique of Functionalist Reason.* Cambridge: Polity Press.

—— (1989) *The New Conservatism: Cultural Criticism and the Historians Debate.* Cambridge: Polity Press.

Illich, I. (1975) *Limits to Medicine. Medical Nemesis: The Expropriation of Health.* Harmondsworth: Penguin.

Lancet (1994) 'Population health looking upstream' (editorial), 343: 429.

—— (1994a) 'US science policy: what science, whose policy?', 343: 367–8.

Marmot, M. and Wilkinson, R. (eds) (1999) *Social Determinants of Health*. Oxford: Oxford University Press.

Merton, R. (1973) *The Sociology of Science*. Chicago, IL: University of Chicago Press.

Navarro, V. (1978) *Class Struggle, the State and Medicine*. London: Martin Robertson.

Pearce, N. and Crawford-Brown, D. (1989) 'Critical discussion in epidemiology: problems with the Popperian approach'. *Journal of Clinical Epidemiology*, 42: 177–84.

Phillimore, P. and Moffatt, S. (1994) 'Discounted knowledge: local experience, environmental pollution and health'. In Popay, J. and Williams, G.H. (eds) *Researching the People's Health*. London: Routledge.

Pill, R. and Stott, N.C. (1985) 'Prevention procedures and practices among working class women: new data and fresh insights'. *Social Science and Medicine*, 21: 975–83.

Platt, S.D., Martin, C.J., Hunt, S.M. and Lewis, C.W. (1989) 'Damp housing, mould growth and symptomatic health state'. *British Medical Journal*, 298: 1673–8.

Popay, J. and Williams, G.H. (eds) (1994) *Researching the People's Health*. London: Routledge.

Popper, K. (1972) *Objective Knowledge*. Oxford: Clarendon Press.

Rice, C. and Roberts, H. (1994) 'It's like teaching your child to swim in a pool full of alligators: lay voices and professional research on child accidents'. In Popay, J. and Williams, G.H. (eds) *Researching the People's Health*. London: Routledge.

Roberts, H. (1994) 'Risk'. *Medical Sociology News*, Winter.

Selborne, D. (1985) *Against Socialist Illusion: A Radical Argument*. London: Macmillan.

Shaw, M., Dorling, D., Gordon, D and Davey Smith, G. (1999) *The Widening Gap: Health Inequalities and Policy in Britain*. Bristol: Policy Press.

Thompson, E.P. (1963) *The Making of the English Working Class*. Harmondsworth: Penguin.

Thompson, E.P. and Yeo, E. (1971) *The Unknown Mayhew: Selections from the Morning Chronicle*. Harmondsworth: Penguin.

—— (1973) *The Unknown Mayhew: Selections from the Morning Chronicle, 1849–50*. Harmondsworth: Penguin.

Trichopoulos, D. (1996) 'The Future of Epidemology', *British Medical Journal*, 313 : 436-7

Watterson, A. (1993) 'Occupational health in the UK Gas Industry'. In Platt, S., Thomas, H., Scott, S. and Williams, G. (eds) *Locating Health. Sociological and Historical Explorations*. Aldershot: Avebury.

Williams, S. and Calnan, M. (1996) *Health and Medicine: Lay Perspective and Experiences*. London: UCL Press.

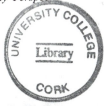

Williams, G.H. and Popay, J. (1994) 'Lay knowledge and the privilege of experience'. In Gabe, J., Kelleher, D. and Williams, G.H. (eds) *Challenging Medicine*. London: Routledge.

Williams, S., Gabe, J. and Calnan, M. (eds) (2000) *Health, Medicine and Society: Key Theories, Future Agendas*. London: Routledge.

Williams, G.H., Popay, J. and Bissell, P. (1997) 'Public health risks in the material world: barriers to social movements in health'. In Gabe, J. (ed.) *Medicine, Health and Risk (Sociology of Health and Illness Monograph)*. Oxford: Blackwell.

Wolfe, T. and Johnson, E.W. (1975) *The New Journalism,* London: Picador.

Zola, I.K. (1972) 'Medicine as an institution of social control'. *Sociological Review*, 20: 487–504.

Chapter 3

System, lifeworld and doctor–patient interaction

Issues of trust in a changing world

Graham Scambler and Nicky Britten

Although by no means the first sociologist to comment on the nature of the relationship between doctors and patients, Parsons' (1951) contribution has long been acknowledged as seminal. By offering a comprehensive, integrated and, above all, *sociological* account of one of the more sensitive, immediate and emblematic of modern relationships – of interest, incidentally, well beyond the formal parameters of his structural-functionalism (Gerhardt, 1987) – he provoked an ever-shifting series of theoretical and empirical studies which shows few signs of abating. Scarcely less influential was Freidson's (1970) critique. Whereas Parsons saw the 'asymmetrical' relationship between doctor and patient – with the doctor characteristically 'active' and the patient characteristically 'passive' – as functionally appropriate, Freidson insisted that the patient too is typically 'active', allowing for a potential *clash of perspectives* between the two parties. Freidson's work precipitated a new interest in, and respect for, a patient's definitions and evaluations of their situations, and how these *lay* constructions might vary independently of the *professional* or *expert*, and culturally authoritative, constructions of doctors.

The pioneering accounts of Parsons and Freidson, together with the programmes of empirical work they rapidly generated, might be described as exemplars of different 'phases' in the development of sociology itself. Referring to British sociology since 1945, Kilminster (1998) has discerned three such phases: the 'monopoly' phase, circa 1945–65; the 'conflict' phase, circa 1965–80; and the 'concentration' phase, circa 1980 to the present. Parsonian theory is of course representative of the structural-functionalist monopoly in British as well as US sociology in the immediate postwar period; and Freidson's *Profession of Medicine* can be interpreted as one product of the conflict phase, which Kilminster defines as one in which advocates of alternate and incommensurable sociological paradigms fight for (monopolistic) supremacy. But what of sociology, and of studies of the doctor–patient relationship over the last two decades, during the so-called concentration phase?

Kilminster insists, plausibly enough, that it is more difficult to specify the contours of the phase through which one is living than it is to be precise about past phases. But he assembles a number of telling observations. Principal among these are his claims that the concentration phase has witnessed a decline in inter-paradigmatic rivalry and partisanship in sociology; that one of the main tensions now is between the 'twin alternatives' of *theoretical synthesis* and *theoretical pluralism*; and that at present 'the longer-term *centripetal* tendency towards *synthesis* just has the upper hand over the *centrifugal* movement towards *fragmentation*' (whereas in the conflict phase 'the balance was tipped the other way') (Kilminster, 1998: 167; original emphasis). Insofar as there is merit in these observations, to what extent do they capture or bear on medical sociology's theorization and study of the doctor–patient relationship?

It must be acknowledged that recent approaches to the doctor–patient relationship – or, increasingly, doctor–patient *interaction* and *communication* – seem characteristic of a new or post-conflict phase: the field is no longer dominated by work within clearly demarcated and contested paradigms. But it is not obvious either that theoretical synthesis has the edge over theoretical pluralism, or that recent studies are more suggestive of centripetal than centrifugal forces. We would emphasize three closely related properties of contemporary investigations.

First, they are for the most part *under-theorized*. In fact, not only are they unlikely to be the issue of discrete and identifiable paradigms (with the exception perhaps of Foucauldian offerings), but their authors seem typically to eschew the generation and testing of substantive sociological theory altogether, in favour of description, of 'typification' or of a (positivist) search for those interactional or communicative 'qualities' of the doctor–patient relationship that are predictive of positive outcomes for health, for future health-related behaviours or for patient satisfaction (see Ong *et al.*, 1995). Second, they tend to present the doctor–patient relationship as an *autonomous or self-contained unit of analysis*, conceptualizing it moreover in terms of a series of independent and 'de-contextualized' encounters (each one displaying an assembly or mix of predefined positive versus negative interactional or communicative characteristics). One consequence of this is that the broader and more sociological – especially macro-sociological – analyses of the doctor–patient relationship that were commonplace during sociology's monopolistic and conflict phases have all but dried up. And third, studies are typically *driven by health policy*. Through the 1990s in Britain and elsewhere (increasingly commissioned) research funding has been made disproportionately available for investigations into ways of enhancing the effectiveness and efficiency of clinical and health promoting interventions, notably in primary care, and this new pragmatism has informed and focused approaches to doctor–patient interaction and communication. It might be argued further, adopting the terminology of Habermas (1984, 1987), that this triad of properties of contemporary studies of the doctor–patient relationship is in part too a function of system rationalization, lifeworld colonization and the binding and inhibiting 'system ties' of many medical sociologists (Scambler, 1996, 1998).

This chapter emphasizes the relevance of sociological theory for understanding the doctor–patient relationship, as well as for analysing face-to-face doctor–patient interaction and communication; and it draws on the varied works of Habermas, as well as on those of other contemporary theorists, to these ends. In the opening section it is argued in general terms that a 'macro'-sociological analysis is as salient and necessary in these contexts as the currently more familiar – and more enthusiastically exhorted and calculatingly sponsored – 'micro'-sociological analyses. In the second section aspects of Habermas' theory of communicative action are summarized and the theory's potential for informing and shaping micro-sociological accounts of different types of encounters and exchanges between doctors and patients explored. An attempt is made here to 'anchor' Habermas' sometimes abstruse and formal theorizing through references to past and present empirical studies. And in the third and final section we maintain that this kind of philosophically and theoretically 'grounded' micro-sociological analysis of doctor–patient relations both requires and lends itself to a complementary macro-sociological analysis of the linkages between these relations and the subsystems of the economy and the state. Attention is paid here to recent explications and theories of 'trust'. Some pointers for generating a credible sociological theory of the doctor–patient relationship which unifies or 'brings together' micro- and macro-sociological accounts are then offered.

Micro- and macro-sociological analyses

C. Wright Mills (1959) was characteristically forthright in his insistence that 'personal troubles' arise in the context of, and must be understood in terms of, social structures.

It is an injunction which has informed the approach to the doctor–patient relationship adopted by Waitzkin (1989, 1991). He notes that, although medical encounters are 'microlevel' processes that involve the interaction of individuals, these processes take place in a context which is shaped by 'macrolevel' social structures. 'Structures of society', he writes, 'help generate the specific social context in which patients and doctors find themselves. The talk that occurs in medical encounters also may reinforce broader social structures' (1989: 221). In a later and more comprehensive treatment of this same theme, Waitzkin offers something akin to a Weberian ideal type of the medical encounter (while readily admitting the existence of 'negative cases'). He is worth quoting at length here:

> ... the theory argues that medical discourse contains an underlying structure, rarely recognized consciously by doctors and patients who speak with each other. In the social contexts of patients' lives, issues arise that create personal troubles. Such issues include difficulties with work, economic insecurity, family life and gender roles, the process of ageing, the patterning of substance use and other 'vices', and resources to deal with emotional distress. To varying degrees during the medical encounter, patients express these troubles. Although some humanistically inclined doctors supportively listen to such concerns, the traditional format of the interview does not facilitate their expression. Countertextual tensions then arise, sometimes manifested at the margins of discourse, or through dominance gestures like interruptions, cut-offs, and de-emphases that move the dialogue back to a technical track. The management of contextual problems involves reified, technical solutions (such as medication) or counselling, but also subtler verbal processes that maintain professional surveillance of individual action and that reproduce mainstream ideologic

assumptions about appropriate behaviour. Medical management also reproduces ideology through crucial absences – for instance, a lack of criticism focusing on social context and an exclusion of such unspoken alternatives as collective action leading to social change. In the process, medical discourse contributes to social control by reinforcing individual accommodation to a generally unchanged context. With the technical help and emotional gratification that they have received, patients perhaps become better equipped to cope, as they continue their consent to the social conditions that troubled them in the first place.

(Waitzkin, 1991: 231–2)

The means Waitzkin deploys to record and reveal the 'structural elements' of medical encounters are of interest (1991: 45–6). In fact, he analyses each encounter in terms of the following:

A) **Social issue as context:** 'social issues' embedded in the economic, social and political dynamics of society often lie behind and help generate the 'personal troubles' that people experience in their day-to-day lives.

B) **Personal trouble:** people tend to experience personal troubles as 'private' or as peculiar to themselves and are unlikely to recognize the social issues that lie behind them.

C) **Medical encounter:** the complaints that people present within medical encounters often, if not always, have contextual sources in, for example, class structure and the organization of work; family life, gender roles and sexuality; ageing and the social role of the elderly; the patterning of leisure and 'substance use'; and limited resources for dealing with emotional distress.

D) **Expression of contextual problems in medical discourse:** the traditional technical sequence of the medical encounter is not conducive to the articulation of contextual concerns; moreover the expression of such concerns is especially difficult for working-class people, women and members of ethnic minorities, and when doctors are neither 'humanistic' nor 'progressive'.

E) **Countertextual tensions deriving from social context:** contextual problems create tensions in medical discourse and occasionally erupt into it, or appear at its margins, and create a 'countertexual reality' that cannot be resolved within the framework of a medical encounter; doctors tend to suppress such tensions by 'dominance gestures like interruptions, cut-offs, and de-emphases that get the discourse back on a technical track'.

F) *Management of contextual problems:* generally contextual problems are converted into technical ones; the status quo is reproduced by accepting the present context as given and rendering social change 'unthinkable', this being medicine's main contribution to social control.

Figure 3.1 demonstrates Waitzkin's use of these categories by summarizing the analysis of a single medical encounter. The encounter involves a 41-year-old man who is described as 'Catholic, black, divorced, a high school graduate, and the father of three children'. He has diabetes, works as an assistant food operations manager in a hotel and is presenting for the first time with pain in his back and neck. This pain worsens with physical movements at work and he finds it difficult to rest at home because of the demands of the job. The doctor, who is described as a '43-year-old white male who practices general internal medicine and endocrinology', and who declares himself to be a Mormon, utlimately prescribes drugs to relieve the pain, a neck collar, heat and other measures to relieve muscle spasm, and advises as much rest as possible. At the core of Waitzkin's analysis is the manner in which the discourse reproduces the ideology of individual responsibility for job-related problems.

Waitzkin's contributions are important: they add up to a compelling case that relationships between doctors and patients can only be comprehensively theorized if they are considered against the background of broader social contexts and structures. But his work remains sociologically unambitious. For all his annotated references to the studies of Marx, Gramsci, Lukács, Althusser and Habermas, his theory retains a rather narrow, orthodox and dated focus on mechanisms of social control. Moreover, there are empirical studies suggesting the need for a more subtle and discriminating theorizing. For example, Gabe and Lipshitz-Phillips (1984) examined the role of tranquillizers in terms of the medicalization of everyday life and the reinforcement of wider hierarchical social relations. They found little evidence that benzodiazepine prescribing and use involved the individualization of social problems or the creation of patient dependence. They also concluded that there was

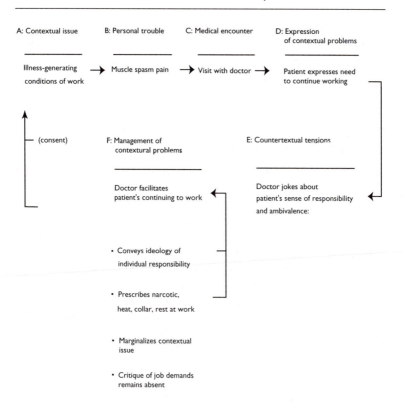

A: Contextual issue   B: Personal trouble   C: Medical encounter   D: Expression
                                                                        of contextual problems

Illness-generating   → Muscle spasm pain → Visit with doctor → Patient expresses need
conditions of work   to continue working

(consent)   F: Management of   E: Countertextual tensions
               contextural problems

               Doctor facilitates   Doctor jokes about
               patient's continuing to work ←   patient's sense of responsibility ←
                                                    and ambivalence:

• Conveys ideology of
  individual responsibility

• Prescribes narcotic,
  heat, collar, rest at work

• Marginalizes contextual
  issue

• Critique of job demands
  remains absent

Figure 3.1   Structural elements of a medical encounter
Source: Waitzkin (1991: 83–92)

a general lack of support for the claim that benzodiazepines served as a form of social control, although this was admittedly based on doctors' claims that they were not influenced by drug companies (a claim exposed as unreliable in other studies (see Avorn *et al.*, 1982)). The authors felt that more sophisticated analyses of the doctor–patient relationship are required, since it is a relationship that contains potentially contradictory elements of differentiation/opposition and association/cooperation, which means that it is at the same time both stratified – in terms of power – and cooperative – in terms of interchange.

It is part of the argument of this chapter that the varied contributions of Habermas have a special, subtle and more flexible potential to re-theorize and illuminate doctor–patient encounters in ways which integrate micro- and macro-perspectives. In the next section the focus is on the relevance of Habermas' work for micro-sociological analyses of the doctor–patient relationship; in the following section the discussion is extended to accommodate macro-analyses.

Doctor–patient encounters: communicative versus strategic action

What Habermas' theory of communicative action does is afford the means to diagnose what Wodak (1996) refers to as 'disorders of discourse'. Since his theory is well known, a brief synthesis oriented to present concerns will suffice. His 'formal pragmatics' provides a suitable starting point. This draws on Austin's (1962) distinction between three types of 'speech act': 'locutionary', 'illocutionary' and 'perlocutionary'. By using locutionary speech acts a speaker says something by expressing a state of affairs. By using illocu-tionary speech acts a speaker performs an action in saying something, generally by means of a performative verb in the first person present (e.g. 'I promise you that "p"'). And by using perlocutionary speech acts a speaker produces an effect on a hearer. Habermas (1984: 288–9) characterizes these three types of speech act in the following 'catchphrases': 'to say *something*, to act *in* saying something, to bring about something *through* acting in saying something'.

For Habermas, 'communicative action' is linguistically mediated interaction in which all speakers pursue illocutionary aims in order to reach 'an agreement that will provide the basis for a consensual coordination of individually pursued plans of action'. 'Strategic action', on the other hand, occurs when at least one speaker aims to produce perlocutionary effects on his/her hearer(s). Perlocutionary effects ensue 'whenever a speaker acts with an orientation to success and thereby instrumentalizes speech acts for purposes that are contingently related to the meaning of what is said' (Habermas, 1984: 289). Communicative action, in short, is oriented to under-standing, and strategic action is oriented to success.

Some elaboration is required at this point. Simple imperatives, like requests or demands, are illocutionary acts with which the speaker 'openly' pursues his/her aim of influencing the hearer(s) (and with which a power claim is associated). In such cases the speaker pursues illocutionary aims unreservedly, but nonetheless acts with an orientation to success rather than understanding. Habermas calls this *open strategic action*. When speakers employ speech acts for perlocutionary ends, this is referred to as *concealed strategic action*. In the case of either open or concealed strategic action 'the potential for the binding (or bonding) force of good reasons – a potential which for Habermas is always contained in linguistic communication – remains unexploited. This potential is only realized in communicative action, when illocutionary acts express *criticizable validity claims*. In the context of communicative action all comprehensible speech acts raise criticizable validity claims concerning truth, appropriateness (or justification) and sincerity. Speakers can 'rationally motivate' hearers to accept their speech acts because they can assume the 'warranty' for providing, if necessary, good reasons that would stand up to hearers' criticisms of validity claims (Scambler, 1987).

Habermas regards what he calls communication 'pathologies' as the result of confusion between actions oriented to understanding and actions oriented to success. Instances of concealed strategic action may involve either conscious or unconscious deception. In cases of conscious deception at least one of the participants acts with an orientation to success, but allows the other(s) to assume that all the conditions of communicative action are being met. This 'manipulation' has been touched on briefly in the discussion of perlocutionary acts. Of unconscious deception, Habermas writes:

> the kind of repression of conflicts that the psychoanalyst explains in terms of defence mechanisms leads to disturbances of communication on both the intrapsychic and interpersonal levels. In such cases at least one of the parties is deceiving himself about the fact that he is acting with an attitude oriented to success and is only keeping up the appearance of communicative action.
>
> (1984: 332)

Habermas refers to unconscious deception as 'systematically distorted communication'. Figure 3.2 (see over) affords a summary of this account.

Habermas' formal pragmatics have a clear relevance for doctor–patient encounters. Doctors have been historically partial to open strategic action; in Britain this has often taken – and still commonly takes – the paternalistic form: 'I'm the doctor, I know

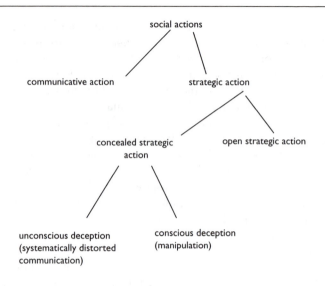

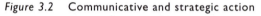

Figure 3.2   Communicative and strategic action
Source: Habermas (1984)

best' (see Graham and Oakley, 1981). As more patient-centred styles of communication have gained ground, emphasizing mutuality and reciprocity, open strategic action has become less acceptable to patients in routine, non-emergency consultations (although it does not follow from this that the potential for a 'clash of perspectives' has in any way diminished). In this altered context, Habermas' analysis of concealed strategic action is particularly useful; and we have seen that this is a concept which covers not only conscious deception, or manipulation, as when a doctor uses technical jargon to browbeat, subdue or gain assent from a resistant patient, but also unconscious deception, or systematically distorted communication, when neither doctor nor patient is aware that strategic rather than communicative action prevails. The concept of systematically distorted communication allows for doctors (not uncommonly) or patients (more rarely) to act with an orientation towards success, not understanding, but yet sincerely and in good faith. This is an issue to which we return below when dealing with trust.

Habermas sees his formal pragmatics as constituting an essential point of departure and 'guide' for empirical-pragmatic investigations, and Mishler (1984) has sought to apply them in this way to episodes of doctor–patient communication. What Mishler calls the *voice of medicine* – its 'legitimacy' underpinned by an expert – and opaque – science-based 'formal knowledge' (Freidson, 1986) – is characterized by strategic action, or action oriented to success: doctors who use the voice of medicine, in short, promote distorted communication by 'leading' patients, consciously or otherwise, towards a particular desired endpoint. While the voice of medicine is not intrinsically problematic, it nevertheless, as an indirect product of what Habermas defines as processes of selective (or excessive system) rationalization and lifeworld colonization, has come to privilege the 'scientific' over what Schutz called the 'natural attitude', even to the extent of medicalizing everyday life (Illich, 1975). As Mishler (1984: 104) observes: 'the meaning of events is provided through abstract rules that serve to decontextualize events, to remove them from personal and social contexts'. When a doctor, wittingly or otherwise, dominates or controls an encounter with a patient this typically has the effect of absorbing and dissolving the patient's self-understanding into a system of purposive-rational action, namely, the framework of technical (bio)medicine. Current clinical practice, Mishler asserts, is based on and incorporates an asymmetrical power relationship between doctor and patient, a view with strong antecedents in sociology's conflict phase but for which there remains a substantial body of support (see, for example, Beisecker, 1990; Maseide, 1991; ten Have, 1991; Brody, 1992). Echoing Freidson rather than Parsons, he continues: 'achieving humane care is dependent upon empowering patients' (Mishler, 1984: 193). In sum, the voice of medicine has developed and retains a tendency to suppress and colonize the *voice of the lifeworld*: lifeworld rationalization and decolonization require patient empowerment.

Mishler argues that if doctors listened more, asked open-ended questions, translated technical language into the voice of the lifeworld and negotiated a sharing of power, they would become not only more humane but more effective practitioners. He developed these ideas out of an analysis of twenty-five consultations in private practice and hospital outpatient departments, a subset of those recorded by Waitzkin and his colleagues (see Waitzkin, 1991). Through the analysis, he discerned a typical mode of communication, the *Unremarkable Interview*. Consultations in this format were conducted wholly in the voice of medicine and showed a uniform structure: first, a request from the doctor; second, a response from the patient; third, a post-response assessment, not always explicit, followed by a new request; and fourth, if optionally, a request for clarification or elaboration of the patient's response. The unremarkable interview, according to Mishler, derives any coherence it might have from the more or less unrestrained dominance of the voice of medicine; but this is accomplished at the cost of the fragmentation, diminution and neglect of the voice of the lifeworld.

The voice of the lifeworld was not entirely missing or without purchase in all twenty-five consultations, but Mishler found that in only one did the doctor actually cede control and opt not to persist with the voice of medicine. He sees this single interview as distinguished by the occurrence of a more humane and effective medicine. His criteria for humane medicine are culled from the American Sociological Association's subcommittee on the humanization of medicine, which commends a view of patients as 'autonomous, unique and irreplaceable "whole persons", who are treated with empathy and warmth and share in decisions with doctors in an equal and egalitarian relationship' (Howard et al., 1977).

Mishler spells out why he regards the unremarkable interview as less than humane and effective:

> the reason is that the voice of medicine relies exclusively on the biomedical model (Mishler, 1981). This model, reflecting the technical-instrumental framework of the biosciences, strips away social contexts of meaning on which a full and adequate understanding of patients and their illnesses depend. Effectiveness of practice depends on such an understanding ... humaneness and effectiveness of care are bound together and do not stand in opposition to each other.
>
> (1984: 192)

This is a strong claim. Moreover it is far from self-evident that a doctor who is less than humane, perhaps due in part to time constraints, cannot be, or rarely is, the agent of effective therapy; or that a humane doctor, perhaps under strict budgetary controls, cannot be, or rarely is, culpable of ineffective therapy. There may well be an empirical association between humaneness and effectiveness, and their combination may be (intrinsically) desirable, but this is not as straightforward a matter as Mishler sometimes implies. Although many patients, for example, resent and are upset by the dominant and colonizing voice of medicine (see, for example, Coyle, 1999), others are content to collude with it (Aronson *et al.*, 1985; Coupland *et al.*, 1994). In a similar vein, Buchanan (1993) found that while most patients with epilepsy were ready to assume responsibility for their anti-epileptic medication, as many as one in four preferred not to do so but simply to 'comply' unquestioningly with the voice of medicine.

In a recent investigation, Barry *et al.* (2000) sought to test Mishler's claim that the dominating voice of medicine equates with inhumane and ineffective care. They analysed thirty-five general practice case studies by means of patient interviews, doctor interviews and transcribed consultations. They found four principal 'communication patterns' across the case-studies: *strictly medicine, mutual lifeworld, lifeworld ignored* and *lifeworld blocked.* The rubric *strictly medicine* was used when doctor and patient both relied exclusively on the voice of medicine, as was typically the case with acute physical complaints; this seemed to work for what the authors describe as 'simple unitary problems'. *Mutual lifeworld* characterized consultations within which both doctor and patient engaged with the lifeworld. These consultations were more relaxed and the voice of the lifeworld was a natural ingredient. They were most common in the context of a combination of psychological and physical problems. The poorest outcomes (measured in terms of ten patient-centred endpoints, such as 'information/reassurance that was required' and 'self-reported adherence') occurred where patients used the voice of the lifeworld but were either ignored (*lifeworld ignored*) or blocked (*lifeworld blocked*) by doctors' use of the voice of medicine. This was most prevalent with chronic physical complaints. The authors conclude that increased use of the voice of the lifeworld does make for better outcomes and more humane treatment. They observe too that doctors seemed able to switch strategies, suggesting their behaviour might be open to change.

The salience of the voice of the lifeworld for effective and humane medical therapy seems clear, as does the propensity for doctors to neglect it in favour of the voice of medicine. What seems no less clear, but has not yet been satisfactorily addressed here, is that the voice of medicine can entirely dominate the voice of the lifeworld, and in a manner suggestive of colonization, in circumstances in which both doctor and patient act in good faith and are content with process and outcome. In our view Habermas' concept of systematically distorted communication might offer more illumination in such circumstances than the offerings of Waitzkin, Mishler and others. And one particularly expedient way of broaching these issues is through the idea of trust.

Trust in doctor–patient encounters

Over the last decade or so the notion of trust has been attracting renewed attention on the part of sociologists. In general, it can be said that this is due to a near-ubiquitous feeling that 'existing bases for social cooperation, solidarity and consensus have been eroded and that there is a need to search for new alternatives' (Misztal, 1996: 3). Certainly the phenomena associated with the present era of 'high' or 'late' modernity, or, for some, of postmodernity, like reflexivity, globalization and risk (Giddens, 1990; Beck, 1992), have brought novel uncertainties and confusion. More specifically, against this same background of change and doubt, commentators have emphasized the significance of trust for post-Fordist economic activities (Sabel, 1989), for the invigoration of civil society (Seligman, 1992), and for face-to-face relations with friends, lovers and family (Giddens, 1991, 1992).

In the medical field, a falling off of trust in doctors has been associated in particular with the growth in consumerism. In an early discussion of the phenomenon of de-professionalization, Haug (1975: 206) takes up this theme and argues that calls for greater public accountability in relation to the professions can be associated with a diminution in the belief that professionals like doctors are 'kindly, concerned and trustworthy'. She cites increased litigation and limits placed on medical experimentation as evidence of this reduction in trust. With regard to the former, she claims that 'patients who sue their doctors obviously have lost trust in them'. And in relation to the latter, she states that 'politicization of the whole experimentation issue is undoubtedly a reflection of public scepticism concerning the researching physician's concern for his patient's welfare. Proof of this concern is required by the regulations, and demands for proof are incompatible with trust. Indeed, trust might be defined as belief without proof.' Roter and Hall (1992) also discuss consumerism in health care. They cite a study carried out by Hibbard and Weeks in 1985 in which 2,000 'consumers' were interviewed to determine the degree to which they behaved as consumers in relation to health care. They found that respondents who reported greater faith in doctors, and more dependence on them, were much less likely to adopt a consumerist orientation.

Misztal attempts a multidimensional definition of trust which is explicitly sociological and which is of relevance to the present focus on the doctor–patient relationship. She argues that trust has many functions:

> it can be a silent background, sustaining unproblematic and smooth-running cooperative relations. It can be a solution of the free-rider problem. It can help people to reconcile their own interests with those of others. It can provide political leaders with the necessary time to carry out reforms. It can offer friends or lovers a platform from which to negotiate their relations. But above all, trust, by keeping our mind open to all evidence, secures communication and dialogue.
>
> (1996: 95)

Misztal seeks an account which allows for this diversity of function. She starts with three assumptions. The first, following Luhmann (1979), is that trust should be understood sociologically in terms of its functions. But whereas Luhmann insists that trust has a single function (namely, to reduce social complexity), Misztal contends that social order requires to be seen not only as a 'stable' system (after Luhmann), but also as a 'cohesive' and 'collaborative' one. Thus trust has functions in relation to each of these three orders.

The second assumption, this time after Giddens (1990), is that there is a connection between inner traits and personal capacity to trust and 'more general trust attitudes'. Giddens (1990: 97) writes: 'trust, ontological security and a feeling of the continuity of things and persons remain closely bound up with one another in the adult personality'. Trust requires not only ontological security but a variety of social forms that provide the conditions 'in which bonds of solidarity can flourish'. And Misztel's third assumption concerns trust's role as a social lubricant, collective good or social capital (see Coleman, 1990; Gambetta, 1988; Putnam, 1993). Returning to the notion of trust's functions in relation to stability, cohesion and collaboration, Misztal (1996: 96) writes: 'we should examine the role of trust relations in stable, cohesive and collaborative orders by asking respectively: how is the stability of social order protected? Whom do we tust? What are the conditions for collaboration?'

In relation to stability, trust is in many ways a device for coping with the contingent and arbitrary in the social world. 'Habitus' is the core concept here. Bourdieu (1977: 72) defines habitus in terms of 'systems of durable, transposable dispositions' which are consequent upon objective structures but capable also of producing and reproducing those structures. Although people internalize 'the immanent law of the structure in the form of habitus', they remain creative within the limits of the structure (Bourdieu, 1992: 98). Drawing an analogy between habitus and trust, Misztal (1996: 98) suggests trust can be seen as a 'system of lasting and transposable dispositions which, integrating past experience, functions at every moment as a matrix of perceptions, appreciation and actions, and makes possible the achievement of (an) infinitely diversified task' (Bourdieu, 1977: 83), endowing the social order with predictability, reliability and legibility. Stability is practically accomplished through 'habit', 'reputation' and 'memory'.

With reference to cohesion, trust is a device to cope with the authenticity of others. The core concept here is 'passion'. Dunn (1993: 641) sees trust in this sense as an 'affective condition, linked to expectations of others' future action'. In Parsonian terms, it is based on others' 'collectivity-orientation'. Cohesion is practically accomplished through 'family', 'friends' and 'society'.

As far as collaboration is concerned, trust is a device for coping with the freedom of others. The core concept here is 'policy'. Its function is to facilitate cooperation. Misztal stresses that trust can only be viewed as a mechanism for solving problems of cooperation when people cooperate independently of the prospect of sanctions or rewards. She draws on Turner's (1989) discussion of the conditions which foster order as cooperative, which she summarizes as follows: 'firstly, it depends on a culturally embedded view of the relationship between self and society (the issue of solidarity). Secondly, it is influenced by the degree of inclusion of individuals and groups to the system (the issue of toleration). Thirdly, the perception of control as non-constraining is shaped by the level of social support for the system and is measured by the degree to which the system is viewed as fair (the issue of legitimacy)' (Misztal, 1996: 99). Collaboration is practically accomplished, then, through 'solidarity', 'toleration' and 'legitimacy'. Misztal's schema is set out in Table 3.1.

What potential does Misztal's articulation of trust have for the sociology of doctor–patient encounters? There are five observations

Table 3.1 Trust: forms and practices

Order	Trust	Practice
Stable	Habitus	Habit Reputation Memory
Cohesive	Passion	Family Friends Society
Collaborative	Policy	Solidarity Toleration Legitimacy

Source: Misztal (1996)

we wish to make. The first builds on the putative links between growing consumerism and declining trust in doctors already broached. It is often asserted that the transition from 'organized' to 'disorganized' capitalism that occurred in the 1960s/1970s embodied a switch of emphasis from 'productivism' to 'consumerism'. Contemporary society, it is frequently said, engages its members primarily in their capacity as consumers rather than producers (see Bauman, 1996). And whereas life organized around the producer's role tends to be 'normatively regulated' (that is, there are both minimum, socially guaranteed levels of well-being, and maximum levels of socially tolerated well-being), life organized around the consumer's role must do without norms: 'it is guided by seduction, ever rising desires and volatile wishes – no longer by normative regulation' (Bauman, 2000: 76). 'Shopping' is the most popular metaphor for consumer society; and, as many now contend, the consumers of disorganized capitalism are inclined to shop around to satisfy their 'desires' and 'wishes' for restored or improved health (or, using the term Bauman (2000) thinks more appropriate to 'postmodern society', 'fitness'). Consumers' shopping around, moreover, increasingly occurs in the 'popular' and 'folk' sectors of what Kleinman (1985) labels 'local health care systems' in addition to the 'professional' sector.

The second point is in a sense a qualification of the first. While there have undoubtedly been changes in the pattern and dynamic of production and consumption over the last generation, it is too easy to ignore their ideological thrust. During his analysis of globalization, Sklair (1998: 140) writes: 'the culture-ideology of consumerism is the fundamental value system that keeps the system intact'; and he continues: 'the point of the concept of the culture-ideology of consumerism is precisely that, under capitalism, the masses cannot be relied upon to keep buying when they have neither spare cash nor access to credit'. In other words, it is essential to recognize that consumerism, including shopping for health (or fitness), is bound up with the mutations of capitalism, and is therefore a likely source of lifeworld colonization. Consumerism, as well as the clientalism now routinely associated with welfare statism, constitutes a threat to citizenship (Hobsbawm, 1999).

The third point concerns the putative shift towards a 'postmodern culture', also dating from the early 1970s. This process of the postmodernization of culture, associated with an emphasis on the 'global' *and* the 'local' (hence Robertson's (1992) coinage of the term 'glocalization'), as well as with a 'disembedding of traditions' (Giddens, 1990), has been accompanied by ubiquitous and virulent forms of relativism. In Lyotard's (1984) phrasing, as the class of 'Grand Narratives' that has been dominant since the European Enlightenment has ceded ground to multiple 'Petit' Narratives, science, including biomedicine, has been 'de-privileged' (some would say 'deconstructed'). It is not of course necessary to subscribe to a postmodern 'reading', or, in Lyotard's case, a celebration of such changes to recognize that they (or something like them) have *in fact* occurred. Doctors have ceased to be the 'legislators' they once were, able unchallenged to prognosticate on matters of health, and instead are taking on the characteristics of 'interpreters' (Bauman, 1987). Drawing on Giddens, Williams and Calnan (1996: 262) note that 'active' forms of trust and 'radical' forms of doubt have become a 'pervasive feature of modern critical reasoning ... all knowledge is tentative, corrigible and therefore open to subsequent revision or abandonment (Giddens, 1991)'. Here, systems of accumulated expertise come to represent multiple sources of authority that are frequently contested and divergent in their implications. Trust, they conclude, 'has *continually* to be "won" and retained in the face of growing doubt and uncertainty (Giddens, 1994)' (emphasis added).

The fourth point concerns the loss of status of doctors over the last generation, not just in Britain but more widely, and possibly gathering momentum through the 1990s.

Discussions of 'proletarianization' and 'de-professionalization', if liable to excess (Elston, 1991), are testimony to this shift in regard. The proletarianization thesis asserts that doctors have become more like other workers, drawn into a factory-like system of production involving a loss of both autonomy and skills. Certainly the 'new managerialism' since the 1980s had something of an equivalent impact. The de-professionalization thesis focuses on the changing relations between doctors and patients. It asserts that the further rationalization of medical knowledge and practice – for example, by means of computerization – and increased lay knowledge about health and disease have undermined the cultural authority of medicine and brought into question its monopoly over health-related knowledge. The public is more critical, it is claimed, of the paternalism of professional experts.

And fifth, reference should be made to the effects on doctor–patient encounters, intended and unintended, of Thatcherite health policy in general and the introduction of the 'internal' or 'quasi-market' into the NHS in 1991 in particular. Gabe and Calnan (2000: 268), noting the change in balance from public to private in the NHS, rightly insist that, although the state remains crucial to the NHS, it is reasonable to suggest that 'the British NHS reflects a new mode of provision – that of the marketized state – and that this set of arrangements has had an effect on the social relations of health care, the manner of its delivery and the experience of consumption'. There is no doubt, for example, that the internal market, and especially GP fundholding, has brought financial considerations into sharper focus. When a primary care centre turns away a family new to the area because of the ramifications of its members' chronic health problems for the centre's budget, or delays hospital referrals until the new financial year, these (potential) patients are much more likely to experience strategic rather than communicative action at the hands of the relevant doctors, either open or, yet more likely, concealed (involving manipulation). Doctors in such cases, it might plausibly be argued, are in a way 'victims' too, any impulse to openness and honesty about financial constraints cut off by the unaccountable bureaucratic instrumentalism of the new managerialism, offspring of the marketized state.

If there is any substance to these five sets of remarks, then it seems undeniable that trust in doctors, in the medical profession, and in medicine itself – in *each* of Misztal's senses, that is, trust as habitus, trust as passion and trust as policy – is every bit as susceptible and threatened in the new era of disorganized capitalism as is the unaccountable and opaque medical paternalism that typified the era of organized capitalism. And it is the basic contention of this chapter that Habermas' theory of communicative action, embodying the dichotomous frame of system/lifeworld and the notions of excessive system rationalization and lifeworld colonization, is an especially promising vehicle for exploring the doctor–patient relationship in general, as well as key issues like the compromising of trust in doctor–patient interaction.

Self-evidently, the construction of a sociological explanation for the kinds of changes to the doctor–patient relationship we have signalled requires a macro- as well as a micro-component. This has long been recognized by authors active in the health domain like Waitzkin; and others, like Mishler, and Barry and her colleagues, have pioneered the empirical application of Habermasian models. This work has prepared the ground for a more sustained theoretical attempt to understand the doctor–patient relationship as related to, and structured by, such macro-phenomena as clientalism and consumerism, themselves aspects of selective rationalization/lifeworld colonization. And it is of course possible, even probable, that processes of clientalism and consumerism might routinely distort doctor–patient interaction and communication despite all parties acting in good faith and with reciprocal satisfaction (Habermas' systematically distorted communication). This chapter represents a tentative and provisional contribution to such a project.

References

Aronson, K., Satterlund Larsson,U. and Saljo, R. (1985) 'Clinical diagnosis and the joint construction of a medical voice'. In Markova, I. and Farr, R. (eds) *Representations of Health, Illness and Handicap*. Switzerland: Harwood Academic Press.

Austin, J. (1962) *How To Do Things With Words*. Oxford: Oxford University Press.

Avorn, J., Chen, M. and Hartley, R. (1982) 'Scientific versus commercial influence on the prescribing behaviour of physicians'. *American Journal of Medicine*, 73: 4–8.

Barry, C., Stevenson, F., Britten, N., Barber, N. and Bradley, C. (2000) 'Giving voice to the lifeworld'. Submitted to *Social Science and Medicine*.

Bauman, Z. (1987) *Legislators and Interpreters: On Modernity, Postmodernity and Intellectuals*. Cambridge: Cambridge University Press.
—— (1996) *Life in Fragments*. Cambridge: Polity Press.
—— (2000) *Liquid Modernity*. Cambridge: Polity Press.
Beck, U. (1992) *Risk Society*. London: Sage.
Beisecker, A. (1990) 'Patient power in doctor–patient communication: what do we know?' *Health Communication*: 105–22.
Bourdieu, P. (1977) *Outline of a Theory of Practice*. Cambridge: Cambridge University Press.
—— (1992) *An Invitation to Reflexive Sociology*. Cambridge: Polity Press.
Brody, H. (1992) *The Healer's Power*. New Haven, CN: Yale University Press.
Buchanan, N. (1993) 'Noncompliance with medication amongst persons attending a tertiary referral epilepsy clinic: implications, management and outcome'. *Seizure*, 2: 79–82.
Coleman, J. (1990) *Foundations of Social Theory*. Cambridge, MA: The Belknap Press of Harvard University Press.
Coupland, J., Robinson, J. and Coupland, N. (1994) 'Frame negotiation in doctor–elderly patient consultations'. *Discourse and Society*, 5: 89–124.
Coyle, J. (1999) 'Exploring the meaning of "dissatisfaction" with health care: the importance of "personal identity threat"'. *Sociology of Health and Illness*, 21: 95–123.
Dunn, J. (1993) 'Trust'. In Goodin, R. and Petit, P. (eds) *A Companion to Contemporary Political Philosophy*. Oxford: Basil Blackwell.
Elston, M. (1991) 'The politics of professional power: medicine in a changing health service'. In Gabe, J., Calnan, M. and Bury, M. (eds) *The Sociology of the Health Service*. London: Routledge.
Freidson, E. (1970) *Profession of Medicine: A Study of the Sociology of Applied Knowledge*. New York: Harper Row.
—— (1986) *Professional Powers: A Study of the Institutionalization of Formal Knowledge*. Chicago, IL: University of Chicago Press.
Gabe, J. and Calnan, M. (2000) 'Health care and consumption'. In Williams, S., Gabe, J. and Calnan, M. (eds) *Health, Medicine and Society: Key Theories, Future Agendas*. London: Routledge.
Gabe, J. and Lipshitz-Phillips, S. (1984) 'Tranquillisers as social control'. *Sociological Review*, 34: 737–72
Gambetta, D. (ed.) (1988) *Trust: Making and Breaking Cooperative Relations*. Oxford: Basil Blackwell.
Gerhardt, U. (1987) 'Parsons, role theory and health interaction'. In Scambler, G. (ed.) *Sociological Theory and Medical Sociology*. London: Tavistock.
Giddens, A. (1990) *The Consequence of Modernity*. Cambridge: Polity Press.
—— (1991) *Modernity and Self-Identity*. Cambridge: Polity Press.

—— (1992) *The Transformation of Intimacy*. Cambridge: Polity Press.

—— (1994) *Beyond Left and Right*. Cambridge: Polity Press.

Graham, H. and Oakley, A. (1981) 'Competing ideologies of reproduction: medical and maternal perspectives on pregnancy'. In Roberts, H. (ed.) *Women, Health and Reproduction*. London: Routledge & Kegan Paul.

Habermas, J. (1984) *The Theory of Communicative Action, Volume One: Reason and the Rationalization of Society*. Cambridge: Polity Press.

—— (1987) *The Theory of Communicative Action, Volume Two: Lifeworld and System: A Critique of Functionalist Reason*. Cambridge: Polity Press.

Haug, M. (1975) 'The deprofessionalization of everyone?' *Sociological Focus*, 8: 197–213.

Hobsbawm, E. (1999) *The New Century*. London: Little, Brown & Co.

Howard, J., Davis, F., Pope, C. and Ruzek, C. (1977) 'Humanizing health care: the implications of technology, centralization, and, medical care'. *Medical Care* (Supplement), 15: 11–26.

Illich, I. (1975) *Limits to Medicine. Medical Nemesis: The Expropriation of Health*. Harmondsworth: Penguin.

Kilminster, R. (1998) *The Sociological Revolution: From the Enlightenment to the Global Age*. London: Routledge.

Kleinman, A. (1985) 'Indigenous systems of healing: questions for professional, popular and folk care'. In Salmon, J. (ed.) *Alternative Medicines: Popular and Policy Perspectives*. London: Tavistock.

Luhmann, N. (1979) *Trust and Power*. Chichester: Wiley.

Lyotard, J.-F. (1984) *The Postmodern Condition*. Manchester: Manchester University Press.

Maseide, P. (1991) 'Possibly abusive, often benign, and always necessary. On power and domination in medical practice'. *Sociology of Health and Illness*: 13.

Mills, C. Wright (1959) *The Sociological Imagination*. New York: Oxford University Press.

Mishler, E. (1981) 'Viewpoint: critical perspectives on the biomedical model'. In Mishler, E., Amara Singham, L., Hauser, S., Liem, S., Osherson, R. and Waxler, N. (eds) *Social Contexts of Health, Illness and Patient Care*. Cambridge: Cambridge University Press.

—— (1984) *The Discourse of Medicine: Dialectics of Medical Interviews*. Norwood, NJ: Ablex.

Misztal, B. (1996) *Trust in Modern Societies*. Cambridge: Polity Press.

Ong, L., de Haes, J., Hoos, A. and Lammes, F. (1995) 'Doctor–patient communication: a review of the literature'. *Social Science and Medicine*, 40: 903–18.

Parsons, T. (1951) *The Social System*. London: Routledge & Kegan Paul.

Putnam, R. (1993) *Making Democracy Work*. Princeton, NJ: Princeton University Press.

Robertson, R. (1992) *Globalization: Social Theory and Global Culture*. London: Sage.

Roter, D. and Hall, J. (1992) *Doctors Talking with Patients, Patients Talking with Doctors: Improving Communication in Medical Visits*. Westport, CN: Auburn House.

Sabel, C. (1989) 'Flexible specialization and the re-emergence of regional economies'. In Hirst, P. (ed.) *Revisiting Industrial Decline*. Oxford: Berg.

Scambler, G. (1987) 'Habermas and the power of medical expertise'. In Scambler, G. (ed.) *Sociological Theory and Medical Sociology*. London: Tavistock.

—— (1996) 'The "project of modernity" and the parameters for a critical sociology: an argument with illustrations from medical sociology'. *Sociology*, 30: 567–81.

—— (1998) 'Medical sociology and modernity: reflections on the public sphere and the roles of intellectuals and social critics'. In Scambler, G. and Higgs, P. (eds) *Modernity, Medicine and Health: Medical Sociology Towards 2000*. London: Routledge.

Seligman, A. (1992) *The Idea of Civil Society*. New York: Free Press.

Sklair, L. (1998) 'The transnationalist capitalist class'. In Carrier, J. and Miller, D. (eds) *Virtualism: A New Political Economy*. Oxford: Berg.

ten Have, P. (1991) 'Talk and institution: a reconsideration of the "asymmetry" of doctor–patient interaction'. In Boden, M. and Zimmerman, D. (eds) *Talk and Social Structure: Studies in Ethnomethodology and Conversation Analysis*. Cambridge: Polity Press.

Turner, R. (1989) 'The paradox of social order'. In Turner, J. (ed.) *Theory Building in Sociology*. London: Sage.

Waitzkin, H. (1989) 'A critical theory of medical discourse: ideology, social control, and the processing of social contexts in medical encounters'. *Journal of Health and Social Behaviour*, 30: 220–39.

—— (1991) *The Politics of Medical Encounters: How Patients and Doctors Deal with Social Problems*. New Haven, CN: Yale University Press.

Williams, S. and Calnan, M. (1996) 'Conclusions: modern medicine and the lay populace in late modernity'. In Williams, S. and Calnan, M. (eds) *Modern Medicine: Lay Perspectives and Experiences*. London: UCL Press.

Wodak, R. (1996) *Disorders of Discourse*. London: Longman

Chapter 4

Health care decision making and the politics of health

Ian Rees Jones

Introduction

Health care decision making is not and cannot ever be value free. By its very nature it is a product of, and acts upon, powerful interests. It cannot escape the consequences of the politics of health. As Paul Atkinson points out: 'Clinical decision making is not the outcome of individual minds, operating in a social vacuum. It is not disinterested, therefore, and is as susceptible to shaping by social influences as any other knowledge' (Atkinson, 1995: 54). In this chapter I will try to address decision making at a number of levels ranging from the micro-decisions that affect individual patients to the public health decision making that reflects the expansive gaze of medical surveillance in today's society. I begin by outlining Habermas' communicative ethics and its relevance to health care. I consider the difficulties this ethics faces when confronted with different understandings of power (particularly medical power). Having set out the theoretical scenery I will address three key areas of health care decision making. First, I will look at changes in the medical encounter. (I will use the term medical encounter throughout this chapter because I am primarily concerned with the doctor–patient relationship and in recent years terms like lay professional relationship and healing relationship have come to the fore partly in recognition of the plastic and open-ended relationships that arise from our increasing concern with health and illness rather than disease.) Secondly, I will examine the rise of managerialism in the NHS, and thirdly I will examine the changing role of public health. Using these exemplars I hope to consider the possibilities and pitfalls of Habermas' project for health care decision making.

Habermas and communicative ethics

Habermas states that linguistic communication between individuals contains implicit 'validity claims' in that what is said is comprehensible, spoken with sincerity, its propositional content is true and it is justified. All of these validity claims are met in the 'ideal speech situation' where there is undistorted communication (Habermas, 1979). Habermas places reliance on truth being achieved through consensus in an ideal speech situation, which is operationalized, by a set of formal rules. The first of these requires that each subject who is capable of speech and action is allowed to participate in discourses. In doing so they are allowed to express their attitudes, wishes and needs. The second requires that they are allowed to introduce any proposal into the discourse and equally may call into question any proposal. The third rule states that these rights to participation should not be proscribed to any speaker by compulsion whether arising from inside or outside the discourse. From these formal rules Habermas proceeds to assert that whoever engages in debate presupposes the validity of the discourse act. Thus, when argumentation concerns norms, the participants implicitly admit that universalization is the only rule under which norms will be taken by all to be legitimate (White, 1988). Norms are the focus for legitimizing the satisfaction of 'human interests' and agreement over a proposed norm should therefore be based on a communicative discourse involving all those affected by the norm. The formal rules for ideal speech do not however constitute a means of producing justified norms, rather they form a procedure for testing the validity of hypothetical norms (Habermas, 1990).

Having set out these formal rules, it seems sensible to ask whether they offer a framework for discussing human interests in an open and fair manner that allows these interests to change and develop in response to open and fair debate. The communicative ethics proposed by Habermas promises fair procedures for judging normative claims but Habermas states that discourses involving experts interpreting the needs of others do not qualify in this respect. The requirements of such an ethics seem to make excessive demands of the actors involved. Actors engaged in discourse are required to be flexible, critical and willing to change their view of needs in response to the discourse. Critics have pointed out that these requirements may be based on a naïve presentation of discursive acts. Fraser (1989) seems to suggest that Habermas is deluding us by underestimating the capacity of language to be used by powerful groups and vested interests to control debates. Habermas has, for example, been criticized for a naïvety towards the operation of power in society and the ways in which power discourses invade all speech situations (Keat, 1981; Lukes, 1982). The danger, for some, is that by separating power relations from communicative relations the theory suggests that power is located in words and not in the institutional context in which they are used (Bourdieu, 1991). Habermas, however, seems to see his theory forming the basis of a critical analysis of communicative practices. In this sense the ideal speech situation is a normative guide rather than a practical reality. The relevance of the Habermasian project to the analysis of health care decision making therefore may not lie in any attempt to operationalize his theory but in its potential as a critical framework – a potential tool to expose systematic distortions, 'ideology' or 'false consciousness'. The aim is to utilize it to provide insights into the distortions of communication by powerful groups (Jones, 1999).

The analysis of speech acts can form a basis for an analysis of power but the methods used may well need to be context dependent. Fairclough, for example, has developed a three-dimensional model for critical discourse analysis based on a circuit of analysis from text to discourse practice to social and cultural practices and back to text (Fairclough, 1992, 1995). Habermas' distinction between communicative action and strategic action can provide the basis for evaluating different speech acts (Habermas, 1984). Communicative action is a form of linguistic interaction where all speech acts contain validity claims concerning comprehensibility, sincerity, truth and justification, which are openly criticizable and discursively redeemable. Strategic action, on the other hand, occurs when at least one of the communicants aims to produce an effect on the others through speech acts. Open strategic action occurs where the speaker's intention to influence the listener(s) is openly declared. Concealed strategic action involves deception. This can be conscious deception whereupon the speaker manipulates the speech act to give the impression of communicative action while pursuing the goal of successfully influencing the listener(s). It can also take the form of unconscious deception, where the speaker engages in self-deception concerning the aims of his/her speech act. Questions follow: how can such forms of deception be assessed and does a claim to be able to assess and identify such speech acts necessarily mean assuming a privileged position? Those who have criticized

Habermas' work have certainly identified just such a danger. However, utilizing the theory to frame a critique of existing speech acts is more akin to using it as an 'ideal type'; an abstract form of speech that can be contrasted with actual forms of speech. Merely outlining its usefulness as an analytical tool would, however, be to understate the importance of Habermas' work. This is because discursive practices are increasingly being seen to have an important role to play in processes of social change (Hastings, 1999). It is unclear at present whether recent social transformations give more than a rhetorical nod towards freer and open communicative practices, but this in itself should be of concern if we are to gain a deeper understanding of the impact of wider social processes on health and illness.

Communicative ethics and health care decision making

What are the consequences of relating Habermas' communicative ethics to health care decision making? If health care decisions become grounded in shared understandings of what is necessary based on procedures that rely on communicative discourses, can this lead to fair and just decision making? Can it, for example, lead to democratic decision making? Can it make the control over the development and use of medical knowledge and medical technologies more transparent and open to question? These issues have been addressed over a number of years by Len Doyal, who has applied his original work on *A Theory of Human Need* (Doyal and Gough, 1991) to health care issues. Doyal and Gough argue that there needs to be clearly informed agreement over the appropriate social policies to satisfy human interests. These questions are confounded by lobbying, conflicts of interest and conflicts between individual, moral and professional interests. Doyal and Gough attempt to tackle these conflicting factors by recourse to communicative practices. Their theory therefore has a substantive and procedural part and they base the procedural half on communicative action being a *prerequisite* to the fair discussion of human needs. Consequently they propose rules for the rational and democratic discussion of needs. These require that all participants possess the best available technical knowledge to address the problem in hand. And disputes about such knowledge have to be resolved by means of communicative practices involving processes that maximize democratic participation (see p. 122 of *A Theory of Human Need* for a full exposition of these rules).

In developing these ideas in relation to health care, Doyal has applied the need for such procedural transparency to the assessment of health care needs, measuring the quality of health care, and to the need for explicit rationing of health services (Doyal, 1992, 1994, 1995, 1997). But does a reliance on communicative action take Habermas' theory a step too far? Can we rely on 'pragmatic rules of truth telling' to address the forces of institutional power, when those forces are producing the 'rhetoric of expert needs discourses' (Fraser, 1981:)? We should not forget that medical paradigms act as a major controlling mechanism for debate (Jones, 1999). Medical paradigms of health and illness can be related to Habermas' three-stage validity analysis where the validity of a statement is justified by claims of truth (concerning the objective world), claims of right-ness (concerning the shared world) or claims of truthfulness (concerning the subjective world). Medical definitions of health and illness are often presented as a claim to truth (saying something about the objective world). However, disease and illness as social constructs are part of the shared world. They involve normative claims that can be challenged and defended on a number of levels. The use of medical knowledge as an objective claim to truth means that it possesses a social currency that can give the illusion of free and open debate. It is the tendency of medical knowledge to 'frame' the debate that problematizes the operationalization of Habermas' theory. In the following section, I will examine these issues in rela-tion to three key areas of health care decision making: the medical encounter; the rise of managerialism; and the changing role of public health. My focus will be on research relating to the British experience.

Changes in the medical encounter

In this section I will focus on decision making in the context of the doctor–patient relationship. There is insufficient space here to discuss the large and increasing body of work addressing medical and clinical encounters. The necessarily sketchy backdrop to this discussion therefore is the recognition that recent social transforma-tions and the rise of consumerism in health care have led to a de-centring of the doctor and problematized more orthodox accounts of the doctor–patient relationship. At the same time the study of medical decision making is becoming an important area for psychologists and specialists in medical informatics whose focus is on the processes of decision making and on the potentiality of computer modelling in medical decision making. This is closely tied to the flowering in recent years of the movement for evidence-based medicine which has been defined as 'the conscientious, explicit, and judicious use of current best evidence in making decisions about the care of individual patients' (Sackett *et al.*, 1996). Atkinson (1995) argues that sociological concerns expand the gaze beyond these primary concerns to look at the *actors* involved, the *settings* in which decisions are made and the *timeframe* of decision making. These concerns remind us that decision making involves a wider social milieu than the simple one doctor–one patient relationship. This is immediately apparent in Atkinson's work on consultant ward rounds, but these insights can be applied to other locations. In general practitioner consultations, for example, it is possible to see that decisions can involve other people in other locations and at other times. The general practitioner might consult partners in the same practice, s/he might discuss the case with other professionals as part of the primary care team. In some instances the consultation may involve translators or advocates or where there is a shortage of such services a member of the patient's family acting as translator. The general practitioner may arrive at a decision over a number of consultations involving a complex process of sharing and revisiting information at different points in time and in different places, for example in the surgery, at the patient's home or over the phone. It seems therefore that the duration of medical decision making in various locations is not bounded by unitary acts and the settings for decision making are not unitary but are diverse and complex. Equally, the patient will make decisions at different times in different locations after consulting with the general practitioner and other people involved including carers, family and friends. The de-centring of the doctor in this decision-making network can be seen in recent calls for shared decision making (of which more later).

In the analysis of his fieldwork among haematologists, Atkinson (1995) attempts to capture the micro-politics of the medical encounter. To do so he starts from the work of Mishler (1984) who identified different *voices* of the medical encounter. For Mishler medical encounters form an asymmetrical relationship where it is possible to distinguish between the voice of medicine and the voice of the lifeworld. The voice of medicine is traditionally seen as the dominant voice in this encounter but Mishler's work seems to undermine this, suggesting that it is the narratives of the patients that are *interrupted* by the voice of medicine. Atkinson takes this as his point of departure from Mishler's work, arguing that the dichotomy between the medical voice and the voice of the lifeworld is too simplistic. Such a critique is perhaps mirrored in the view that making an over-rigid distinction between lifeworld and system-world can lead to exaggerated versions of the medicalization thesis. Instead, Atkinson argues that medicine has several voices which co-exist and sometimes come into conflict. Among these he identifies the voice of *experience*, voices of *textbook science* and *journal science*, the voice of *seniority* and the voice of *reminiscence*. The subtle interplay between these different voices during medical encounters is elegantly demonstrated by Atkinson's example of a clinician discussing a case and recounting his involvement in the death of a famous film star (Atkinson, 1995: 138). Atkinson shows us how knowledge is produced and reproduced in micro-settings and how these micro-settings can involve a variety of voices at different times. Medical knowledge and power is orally transmitted in different ways with individuals invoking science, seniority, experi-ence and personal anecdotes at different points in the discourse. While clinicians engage in the use of subtle linguistic codes to express doubt and uncertainty, the use of personal anecdotes, narratives, reminiscences and maxims is particularly related to what Atkinson calls *apodictic* or clearly established knowledge. This anal-ysis suggests a process by which a technical language and linguistic/non-linguistic codes are learnt and passed on by profes-sionals. This process contributes to the manufacture of a monopoly of knowledge and reinforces the 'competence gap' between profes-sional and patient. As Turner (1995) points out, one of the ways the doctor–patient relationship can be examined is by looking at the ways in which this 'competence gap' is filled by distorted communi-cation.

There have been increasing calls in recent years for greater patient participation in health care decision making. Indeed the World Health Organization (WHO) has stated that patient involve-ment in health care decision making is a social, economic and technical necessity (Waterworth and Luker, 1990). Although the evaluation of patient participation in health care decision making is in its infancy (DeMaio, 1993), there is evidence to suggest that there have been policy shifts designed to democratize the medical encounter. The concordance model of the patient–doctor relationship for example was proposed by a national working party of The Royal Pharmaceutical Society of Great Britain. Concordance is a term that is being promoted as a replacement for terms such as patient compliance. It is based on the idea of giving mutual respect to the health beliefs of doctor and patient. The role of medical science here is not seen as one of applying superior knowledge but as a component part of a process where the patient becomes central to both decision making and the practice of health care. These ideas have filtered up to policy initiatives that make a strong distinction between the involvement of people at the level of individual treatment and care and the level of service development (the level of citizens and communities). Clearly there are formal attempts to make public participation a priority (NHS, 1996, 1997). There is, however, very little evidence to show the most effective ways of enhancing patient choice and patient participation (Calnan *et al.*, 1998) and attempts to develop strategies for user involvement in health care decision making are thin on the ground (Kelson, 1995, 1997). Recently there has been a growing interest in shared decision making (Coulter, 1997). Shared decision making requires a process that approaches a symmetrical relationship between health professional and patients. Coulter argues that this could increase the effectiveness of a range of treatments through improvements in information and knowledge on both sides. One of the ways in which this could be achieved is by means of improved information to patients, but a recent review of information materials found the quality of patient material in Britain to be variable and in some cases materials were found to be 'patronizing, victim blaming, dismissive and promoting an attitude of "doctor knows best"' (Coulter *et al.*, 1999). The researchers called for resources to be committed to the development of patient information and the training of clinicians in communications skills. It would be prudent however to retain a sceptical stance towards shared decision making. As Lupton points out, doctor–patient relationships are often ambivalent and relational (Lupton, 1997). It is possible to view the proliferation of patient information as part of a magnification of the medical gaze and an extension of biomedical power. Some recent research suggests that patients want to be involved in decision making but little is known about the ways in which they can become more involved and even less is known about the benefits of their involvement (Guadagnoli and Ward, 1998). Some work has been undertaken on user perceptions of treatments that are rationed in the NHS (Joule, 1998) and this has identified a need for clarity on patients' rights, for openness and honesty with patients and for greater patient participation in decision making.

Forde-Roberts (1998) makes a useful distinction between public and private participation. *Private* participation refers to the involvement of individuals in their own care and treatment. This can lead to increasing patient involvement, more commitment to health and health-promoting behaviours, the development of an ecological concept of health and the improved use of health services (McEwen *et al.*, 1983). On the other hand, participation could lead to a delay in seeking care, risks of conflicting advice, misuse of technical information and the alienation of professionals. *Public* participation refers to taking part in decision-making processes concerning service planning and delivery, service evaluations and consultations over future service provision. It refers to a democratization of decision making, with the public assuming greater responsibility for decisions regarding the wider aspects of health and social policy. Such participation can take place at a number of levels. For example, Arnstein's 'ladder of citizen participation' (Arnstein, 1969) involves eight stages, starting from non-participation and progressing to citizen control. The benefits of public participation depend crucially on the pattern of re-distribution of power. The dangers and risks are that consultation becomes the norm and in the name of participation this is little more than 'tokenism' or 'window dressing' (Biehal, 1993). The increasing concerns about participation at a *micro-level* can be related to the emphasis Habermas places on the role of discourse ethics (Habermas, 1993) in acting as a procedure for open decision making – a means to a solution rather than a solution in itself. At a *macro-level* his argument for a 'deliberative democracy' based on broad popular participation could be construed as being over-reliant on the role of legislature in expressing and formalizing democratic processes but has important implications for attempts to increase patient participation within a closed state institution such as the NHS. Habermas' concern has been with those structural and cultural factors that act as constraints on individual rationality. The inequalities and asymmetries of power in the doctor–patient relationship can be evaluated critically using Habermas' work as a guide but, as Turner (1995) points out, changes in this relationship are dependent on macro-sociological changes and not just on strategies to re-educate doctors and patients.

The rise of managerialism in the NHS

As was mentioned earlier, shifts towards consumerism in health care and a de-centring of doctors in the medical encounter are closely related. But the shift away from doctors is not necessarily a shift towards the patient. Atkinson reminds us that decision-making processes are complex, multifaceted and clearly tied to different notions of status and expertise. Consumerism, on the other hand, introduces new asymmetries while reinforcing others. It is here perhaps that links can be made to the increasing power of managers in health service provision and health service decision making.

Since the publication of the Griffiths Report in 1983 (Griffiths, 1983), the NHS has been following a path towards increasing managerialism. The journey has involved various excursions into resource management initiatives, a headlong rush into internal market in the early 1990s and a tentative withdrawal following the Labour administration of 1997. The trend towards managerialism has coincided with considerable structural and cultural changes that are characterized by greater rationality and efficiency. Efficiency fetishisms in welfare provision have been criticized from a philosophical position (Goodin, 1988), but it is also possible to draw on more pragmatic critiques of these trends. Some attention has been paid to managerial discourses and their relationship to change in the NHS (Traynor, 1996; Hughes, 1996; Harrison and Pollitt, 1994). These writers have highlighted the difference between managerialism as a challenge to professional interests and trends towards incorporating professionals into management roles, the latter perhaps being seen as an alternative to cruder strategies of attempting to control professionals. Traynor (1996) argues that the structure of language reflects existing power relations. Utilizing a Foucauldian approach as a basis for analysing managerial discourses as text (attempting to set aside the intention of speakers), he identifies an emphasis on rationality that draws legitimacy from reference to a capacity for *measurement* and *financial constraint*. Tracing a lineage from Taylorism to Fordism and post-Fordism, Traynor shows how managers make claims to moral neutrality, objectivity and scientific rationalism. The claims made for such capacities allow managers to take up positions of neutrality, to appear as disembodied decision makers whose decisions have natural, logical and inescapable trajectories. Thus such notions of neutrality and objectivity conceal what is essentially political decision making. The consequence in Traynor's eyes is that there is a privileging of measurement. He refers to the work of MacIntyre (1985) to describe a masquerade of managerial capability. Similarly, in his work on culture management, Hughes (1996) notes the 'wily' rhetorical skills that managers deploy in the furtherance of particular interests and agendas. The importance of such rhetorical skills for micro-political struggles has been examined using a Habermasian framework by Forester (1992), who highlights how day-to-day negotiations contain validity claims (claims to truth) that are translated into practical action. The extent to which the structure of language reflects micro-power relations is evident in my own work on the debates among clinicians and managers who were rationalizing health services in London (Jones, 1999). Here the emerging 'internal health care market' in the early 1990s was promoted by managers as something that would improve services, bring about efficiency and enhance consumer choice. But in drawing up a plan to rationalize services these same managers were engaging with clinicians in a task that bypassed the mechanisms of the market to produce a comprehensive rational plan for London's services. Clinicians in particular were uncomfortable with the contradictions that seemed to rise from this. The 'market' meant different things at different times and managers appeared more comfortable with the ambiguities involved. For example, one manager attempted to address the ambiguities by stating:

> ... we do not have a mature balanced market. Our job is first of all to put that in place instead of something unbalanced ...
>
> (Jones, 1999: 109)

Not all the participants in this debate had access to the same 'knowledge' as the managers involved. But instead of sharing their knowledge of markets or acknowledging their own uncertainties, the managers involved seemed more concerned with deploying a smoke screen of jargon and rhetoric. This, it can be argued, involved both conscious and unconscious deception, in that managers were giving the impression of trying to engage in debate while concealing the contradictory nature of their arguments. The fluidity of their position was brought into focus by the possibility that managers were deceiving themselves with these arguments. The use of a technical language by the managers in a form of strategic action is apparent in the following extract where a manager relates how the market can deliver change and how this can be monitored:

> one has to use various efficiency or other terminology to find a way which can demonstrate you've improved local health care year on year.
>
> (Jones, 1999: 108)

The shift from the reciprocal pronoun at the beginning of this sentence to the personal pronoun is important because it gives an indication of how the manager viewed efficiency terminology (reciprocal and abstract) in relation to improvements in local health care (personal). The implication is that efficiency is an objective concept, about which truth claims can be made, while 'demonstrating improvements in local health care' is closer to the manager's personal objectives. Here we see how the language of the market lends itself to a discourse that is removed from reality. The concerns expressed here are less to do with the impact of change on services and patients, but with a discourse that legitimizes the market, and the manager's own position. This can be interpreted as a form of concealed strategic action that involves conscious and unconscious deception. There are other ways of interpreting these speech acts but a Habermasian perspective does, I think, provide another means of exploring particular communicative practices and exposing them to critical evaluation and examination. The challenge seems to be to examine the extent to which such speech acts have become the 'norm' in health service debates, to what extent they represent a further form of system world colonization and/or to what extent they represent a high water mark of market-based rhetoric.

The changing role of public health

Over the last 150 years, public health in Britain has undergone successive transformations. Goraya and Scambler (1998) have chartered these changes from the early *sanitary* phase lasting from about 1840 to 1870, through the *preventative* phase (around 1870), into the *therapeutic* phase lasting from around 1940 until the early 1970s when the prevailing biomedical view of health and disease began to be challenged by the *new public health*. This new public health embodied in the work 'Health for All' and 'Healthy Cities' operates both outside and within mainstream public health institutions (Ashton, 1992). Its aim is to change priorities by developing public health decision making based on strategies of prevention and health promotion. In this sense it differs from the old sanitary public health in its political and ideological dimensions. It has been seen by some as a form of 'new social movement' corresponding with Habermas' view of emancipatory social movements (Milewa and de Leeuw, 1996). Others have seen postmodern tendencies in the plurality of issues, the recognition of difference and the fragmented approach to power (Kelly *et al.*, 1993).

These transformations have consequences for health care decision making in a number of interconnecting fields. Armstrong (1995) has argued that the extension of the medical gaze into communities is a defining characteristic of late modern societies. The suggestion is that this medical gaze provides new data to inform public health decision making while at the same time extending the surveillance of medicine over whole communities. This same process could be described as an extension of the systematizing tendencies of medicine. This problematizes public health because it suggests that the knowledge base for much public health decision making is based on an imperative that contains contradictions (Lupton, 1995). These contradictions can be dissected from a number of perspectives. Some have argued that the epistemological foundations of people's everyday knowledge mean that claims for the 'objectivity' of expert knowledge are contestable. From this perspective, lay knowledge offers a political challenge to the authority of professionals to determine the way in which questions are framed, problems are defined and knowledge produced and reproduced (Williams and Popay, 1994). With respect to public health decision making, an important question therefore is to what extent problems and their solutions are based in available technical knowledge as opposed to the people those decisions affect. Public health experts facing the challenge of addressing health concerns of different communities may find themselves caught in a 'location paradox', trapped between the rationality of the system-world and the experiential nature of lay knowledge (Scambler and Goraya, 1994). The contradictory nature of public health therefore goes beyond surveillance of 'passive' bodies or communities and can be seen in the contrast between the distinct policy ontologies at the centre of emancipatory health policy movements such as 'Healthy Cities' and existing policy ontologies (Milewa and de Leeuw, 1996). Addressing the new urban public health movement Milewa and de Leeuw identify three areas of ontological and communicative conflict. They begin by focusing on *health* and the emphasis that the new public health places on 'equity' and the idea of health as instrumental to other needs. Here they see a direct challenge to orthodox causal links that are made using epidemiology and medical evidence. They then consider *empowerment* and identify a tension between the promotion of individual consumers of health care and a rejection of consumerism in health care. Finally, they identify cultural settings of *community mobilization*, which by their nature can involve exclusion of some communities and groups. The closer organizations get to citizen groups and community groups the more likely they are to be challenged by lifeworld discourses. At the same time bureaucracies may develop a capacity to de-linguify communication and thus resist or even become immune to demands for change. In response to this Milewa and de Leeuw have called for another strategy based on the diffusion of communicative practices, arguing that it is through the acceptance of communicative practices that the metaphors and parameters that exist within dominant policy ontologies can be challenged. The problem with such strategies is their one-sided nature. Indeed, Jackson (1999) questions whether systems can be 'opened up' to the lifeworld within such formal settings. There is a danger that they become concerned with equal distributions of discourse rather than equal distributions of resources. Movements for change can, it seems, be caught up in webs of rhetoric. It is useful I think to look at change at different levels. Scambler and Goraya (1994) identify *operational change* such as formal health promotion work which neither threatens nor challenges core institutions, *political change* which usually requires government action and can pose a threat to institutions and *structural change* which requires mass public support and extra parliamentary political action. Much of existing public health decision making and action still operates at the level of operational change. It may stray within the sphere of political change but its relationship with the sphere of structural change is very much a rhetorical one. If, as Habermas suggests, a deliberative democracy needs mechanisms to de-colonize the lifeworld and to transform lifeworld discourse into administrative power, then the role of the new public health as such a mechanism seems questionable and confused.

Conclusion

Using primarily a British perspective this chapter has looked at changes in health care decision making in a number of different locations. The value of a number of key features of Habermas' work has been explored at a number of different levels and it has been suggested that his theory of communicative action can act as a framework for a critical analysis of decision making. More importantly his influence can be detected in the impetus for more democratic decision making in the locations discussed here and in many others not yet discussed. In this way Habermas' work cannot be seen as purely abstract; it also has practical consequences. His work on the public sphere is particularly relevant to our understanding of health care decision making and the politics of health. To begin with, because of his previous emphasis on the emancipatory potential of new social movements, there is scope for examining the relationship between these movements and challenges to biomedicine. Following on from this, there is a tendency in health and social policy to focus on the communicative practices of particular institutions without taking account of the impact of wider social processes on those practices. Habermas' work on the re-feudalization of the public sphere and the emphasis he gives to the power of the press in influencing public debate is an important counterweight to this. Finally, his call for a deliberative democracy gives weight to the law as a vehicle for transferring citizen needs into administrative power. He appears to envisage a circuit between the public sphere and the government sphere where communicative power is transformed into administrative power. Here the key and perhaps ambivalent role of public health practitioners as decision makers and mediators is worthy of further research. As I stated at the outset, health and health care cannot be reduced to technical considerations of measurement and evaluation. They are a fundamental part of the lifeworld/system-world problematic, and as such are profoundly political. This discussion has only scratched the surface and can be criticized for only asserting the applicability of Habermas' work to health care decision making rather than demonstrating its practical application. Nevertheless, I hope it has opened up a space for furthering our understanding of health care decision making and the politics of health

References

Armstrong, D. (1995) 'The rise of surveillance medicine'. *Sociology of Health and Illness*, 17, 3: 393–404.

Arnstein, S. (1969) 'A ladder of citizen participation'. *Journal of the American Institute of Planners*, 35: 216–24.

Ashton, J. (1992) 'The origin of healthy cities'. In Ashton, J. (ed.) *Healthy Cities*. Milton Keynes: Open University Press.

Atkinson, P. (1995) *Medical Talk and Medical Work*. London: Sage.

Biehal, N. (1993) 'Changing Practice'. *British Journal of Social Work*, 23: 443–58.

Bourdieu, P. (1991) *Language and Symbolic Power*. Cambridge: Polity Press.

Calnan, M., Halik, J. and Sabbat, J. (1998) 'Citizen participation and patient choice in health reform'. In Saltman, R.E., Figueras, J. and Sakellarides, C. (eds) *Critical Challenges for Health Care Reform in Europe*. Buckingham: Open University Press.

Coulter, A. (1997) 'Partnership with patients: the pros and cons of shared clinical decision making'. *Journal of Health Services Research and Policy*, 2: 112–21.

Coulter, A., Entwistle, V. and Gilbert, D. (1999) 'Sharing decisions with patients: is the information good enough?' *British Medical Journal*, 318: 318–22.

DeMaio, S. (1993) 'Lay participation in health care decision making'. *Journal of Health Politics Policy and Law*, 18, 4: 881–904.

Doyal, L. (1992) 'Need for moral audit in evaluating quality in health care'. *Quality in Health Care*, 1: 178–83.

—— (1994) 'Needs, rights and the moral duties of clinicians'. In Gillon, R. (ed.) *Principles of Health Care Ethics*. Chichester: Wiley.

—— (1995) 'Needs, rights and equity: moral quality in health care rationing'. *Quality in Health Care*, 4: 273–83.

—— (1997) 'The rationing debate: rationing within the NHS should be explicit: the case for'. *British Medical Journal*, 314: 1114.

Doyal, L. and Gough, I. (1991) *A Theory of Human Need*. London: Macmillan.

Fairclough, N. (1992) *Discourse and Social Change*. Cambridge: Polity Press.

—— (1995) *Critical Discourse Analysis*. Harlow: Longman.

Forde-Roberts, V.J. (1998) 'Working for patients? An analysis of some effects of the National Health Service reforms in South Buckinghamshire'. Unpublished PhD thesis, Queen Mary and Westfield College, University of London.

Forester, J. (1992) 'Critical ethnography: on fieldwork in a Habermasian way'. In Alverson, M. and Wilmott, H. (eds) *Critical Management Studies*. Newbury Park, CA: Sage.

Fraser, N. (1981) 'Foucault on modern power: empirical insights and normative confusions'. *Praxis International*, 1: 283.

—— (1989) *Unruly Practices, Power Discourse and Gender in Contemporary Social Theory*. Cambridge: Polity Press.

Goodin, R.E. (1988) *Reasons for Welfare: The Political Theory of the Welfare State*. Princeton, NJ: Princeton University Press.

Goraya, A. and Scambler, G. (1998) 'From old to new public health: role tensions and contradictions'. *Critical Public Health*, 8, 2: 141–51.

Griffiths, R. (1983) *NHS Management Enquiry Report*. London: DHSS.

Guadagnoli, E. and Ward, P. (1998) 'Patient participation in decision making'. *Social Science and Medicine*, 47, 3: 329–39.

Habermas, J. (1979) *Communication and the Evolution of Society*. London: Heinemann.

—— (1984) *The Theory of Communicative Action, Volume One: Reason and the Rationalization of Society*. London: Heinemann.

—— (1990) *Moral Consciousness and Communicative Action*. Cambridge: Polity Press.

—— (1993) *Justification and Application: Remarks on Discourse Ethics*. Cambridge: Polity Press.

Harrison, S. and Pollitt, C. (1994) *Controlling Health Professionals: The Future of Work and Organization in the NHS*. Buckingham: Open University Press.

Hastings, A. (1999) 'Discourse and urban change: introduction to this special issue'. *Urban Studies*, 36, 1: 7–12.

Hughes, D. (1996) 'NHS managers as rhetoricians: a case of culture management?' *Sociology of Health and Illness*, 18, 3: 291–314.

Jackson, N. (1999) 'The council tenant's forum: a liminal public space between lifeworld and system?' *Urban Studies*, 36, 1: 43–58.

Jones, I.R. (1999) *Professional Power and the Need for Health Care*. Aldershot: Ashgate.

Joule, N. (1998) *Rationing by Denial? Report of a College of Health Project on User Perceptions of Treatment Subject to Formal Prioritisation in the NHS*. London: College of Health.

Keat, R. (1981) *The Politics of Social Theory*. Oxford: Blackwell.

Kelly, M.K., Davies, J.K. and Charlton, B.G. (1993) 'Healthy cities, a modern problem or a post-modern solution?' In Davies, J.K. and Kelly, M.K. (eds) *Healthy Cities, Research and Practice*. London: Routledge, pp. 159–67.

Kelson, M. (1995) *Consumer Involvement in Clinical Audit and Outcomes*. London: College of Health.

—— (1997) *User Involvement: A Guide to Developing Effective User Involvement Strategies in the NHS*. London: College of Health.

Lukes, S. (1982) 'Of gods and demons: Habermas and practical reason'. In Thompson, J. and Held, D. (eds) *Habermas*. London: Macmillan.

Lupton, D. (1995) *The Imperative of Health: Public Health and the Regulated Body*. London: Sage.

—— (1997) 'Foucault and the medicalisation critique'. In Petersen, A. and Bunton, R. (eds) *Foucault, Health and Medicine*. London: Routledge.

MacIntyre, A. (1985) *After Virtue. A Study in Moral Theory*. London: Duckworth.

McEwen, J., Martini, C.J.M. and Wilkins, N. (1983) *Participation in Health*. London: Croom Helm.

Milewa, T. and de Leeuw, E. (1996) 'Reason and protest in the new urban public health movement: an observation on the sociological analysis of political discourse in the "healthy city"'. *British Journal of Sociology*, 47, 4: 657–70.

Mishler, E. (1984) *The Discourse of Medicine: Dialectics of Medical Interviews*. Norwood, NJ: Ablex.

National Health Service (1996) *Patient Partnership Strategy*. London: NHS Executive Department of Health.

—— (1997) *The New NHS: Modern, Dependable*. London: HMSO.

Sackett, D.L., Rosenberg, W.M.C., Gray, J.A.M., Haynes, R.B. and Richardson, W.S. (1996) 'Evidence based medicine: what it is and what it isn't'. *British Medical Journal*, 312: 71–2.

Scambler, G. and Goraya, A. (1994) 'Movements for change: the new public health agenda'. *Critical Public Health*, 5, 2: 4–10.

Traynor, M. (1996) 'A literary approach to managerial discourse after the NHS reforms'. *Sociology of Health and Illness*, 18, 3: 315–40.

Turner, B.S. (1995) *Medical Power and Social Knowledge* (second edition). London: Sage.

Waterworth, S. and Luker, K.A. (1990) 'Reluctant collaborators. Do patients want to be involved in decisions concerning care?' *Journal of Advanced Nursing*, 15: 971–6.

White, S.K. (1988) *The Recent Work of Jürgen Habermas: Reason, Justice and Modernity*. Cambridge: Cambridge University Press.

Williams, G. and Popay, J. (1994) 'Researching the people's health: dilemmas and opportunities for social scientists'. In Popay, J. and Williams, G. (eds) *Researching the People's Health*. London: Routledge.

Chapter 5

Class, power and the durability of health inequalities

Graham Scambler

Within medical sociology in Britain the continuing existence of what are sometimes referred to as 'health variations' is uncontroversial. Scarcely more so is the significance of social class as *a*, if perhaps no longer *the*, key underlying source of these variations or, as they were formerly and will here be designated, 'inequalities'. By and large, studies into health inequalities involving medical sociologists have been conducted within a particular, dominant paradigm or research programme which can be broadly characterized as *positivist* as defined, for example, by Giddens (1974), accommodating some cautious and thoughtful empirical as well as crassly empiricist work. It has been argued elsewhere that the dominance of this programme of research, and its seductiveness to medical sociologists, has led to the under-development or neglect of a more genuinely sociological and theoretical engagement with the issues, including a failure to take social class seriously as a phenomenon in its own right (Higgs and Scambler, 1998).

The conceptual and theoretical focus of this chapter is one substantive conjecture: namely, that central to any satisfactory sociological analysis of the production, reproduction and failures of social and health policies to reduce health inequalities in the UK is an appreciation of the signal and defining impact of a 'power elite' at the centre of the apparatus of the state, infused as it is by members of what Clement and Myles (1997) call the 'capitalist-executive'. More specifically, what will hereafter be referred to as the 'greedy bastards hypothesis' (GBH) states that health inequalities in the UK can reasonably be interpreted as indirect (and largely unintended) consequences of the ever-adaptive behaviours of members of Britain's power elite and capitalist-executive.

In the opening section of this chapter a brief critical reference to positivist research on class and health inequalities is made. This is succeeded by a succinct rehearsal of an alternative and more unequivocally sociological and theorized approach to the investigation of linkages between class relations and health inequalities, drawing on the works of Bhaskar (1989) and of Clement and Myles (1997) and spelled out more comprehensively elsewhere (see Scambler and Higgs, 1999).

The second section takes its departure from a critical account of Habermas' reconstruction of Marx's theory of class relations which aspires to distinguish between defensible revision and premature displacement. It is maintained that although there is much to commend Habermas' analysis of the uncoupling of system and life-world and of the selective nature of societal rationalization into high modernity, he has too hastily discarded a Marxian insistence on the continuing significance of relations of class.

In the third section the GBH is explicated in some detail, and the fourth and final section builds on previous publications to explore the nature of the hypothesized linkages between the power elite and capitalist-executive and health inequalities. An agenda for future research, conceptual and theoretical as well as methodological, is tentatively suggested. Consideration is given here too to the very real obstacles to making significant progress in empirical research in the near future.

Positivism, health inequalities and re-theorizing class

An ailing paradigm

It is in many respects surprising that positivist research has so effectively survived the scathing critiques of a generation ago. In health inequalities research, it seems, it has not only survived but flourished. Arguably this has a lot to do with both the lead taken by social epidemiologists and statisticians and the micro-politics of the major funding outlets and of academic career-building. While the crudest forms of 'systematic empiricism' tend nowadays to be eschewed within medical sociology (see Willer and Willer, 1973), it remains the case that in the majority of studies on class and health inequalities in which medical sociologists are involved there is disconcertingly little interplay or dialectic between theory and observation. It is not of course that theory is absent from positivist studies; rather, as Johnson and colleagues (1984: 390) insist in respect of equivalent research on the causes of suicide, the decision to incorporate some 'variables' while omitting others 'ultimately depends on some *ad hoc* appeal to, or unstated acceptance of, theoretical ideas'. The presence or acceptance of any theoretical impetus is unacknowledged and fortuitous. Nor is it the case that there is no worthwhile return, even for medical sociology, from positivist research. But in light of critiques produced almost *ad nauseam* in the 1960s, it is probably not overstating things to suggest that an enduring commitment to positivism in medical sociology suggests a worryingly innocent, inefficient and irresponsible use of effort and resources.

There is no need here to provide another review of positivist research on class and health inequalities. Efficient and up-to-date summaries and discussions of this body of research (and more) can be found in many places, including the following triad of volumes. First, the Office for National Statistics has collated the most recent set of nationwide data in the fifteenth decennial supplement (see Drever and Whitehead, 1997). Second, the *Report of the Independent Inquiry into Inequalities in Health* (chaired by Acheson) (Stationery Office, 1998) contains both a wide-ranging research review and a series of recommendations for policy changes with apparent promise for accomplishing greater equality. And, third, a collection of academic papers sponsored by the editorial board of *Sociology of Health and Illness* offers appraisals and exemplars of some current – sophisticated but mainly positivist – programmes of research (as well as some minority non-positivistic comment); tellingly, neither Marx nor (even) Weber figure in the book's index (Bartley *et al.*, 1998).

Positivist studies of health inequalities deploying class as one of a number of 'variables' typically seek to *explain class away* by means of statistical manoeuvres featuring putative 'class-constitutive' or 'class-associated' factors such as educational attainment, properties of work, household income, housing tenure, car ownership and patterns of lifestyle and behaviour. There is a strong case for sociologists rediscovering past ambitions and treating class not merely as one variable among others but as a *phenomenon or object in its own right*. Indeed, it can be argued that, if positivist research on class and enduring health and other forms of social inequalities (see Adonis and Pollard, 1997) has established anything, it is that there must exist real relations of class hinging on the ownership and/or control of the means of production (Higgs and Scambler, 1998; Scambler and Higgs, 1999).

Re-theorizing class relations

The philosophical investigations of Bhaskar underpin the account of real relations of class to be outlined here. Bhaskar (1989) postulates a real ontological difference between *people* and *society*, defining the latter, after Marx, in terms of a 'network or relations': 'people are not relations, societies are not conscious agents' (Collier, 1994: 147). 'Society', Bhaskar (1989: 34–5) writes, 'is both the ever-present *condition* (material cause) and the continually reproduced *outcome* of human agency' (original emphasis). People do not work to produce the capitalist economy any more than they marry to sustain the nuclear family, 'yet it is nevertheless the unintended consequence (and inexorable result) of, as it is also a necessary condition for, their activity. Moreover, when social forms change, the explanation will not normally lie in the desires of agents to change them that way, though as a very important theoretical and political limit, it may do so' (Bhaskar, 1989: 35).

Society as the condition of action and society as its outcome both belong to the subject matter of sociology. And society as an object of inquiry is necessarily 'theoretical' in the sense that it is necessarily unperceivable: it cannot be empirically identified independently of its effects. In this respect it is no different from many of the objects of natural scientific enquiry. Where it does differ, however, is that it not only cannot be empirically identified independently of its effects, but it does not *exist* independently of them either (Bhaskar, 1989a: 82). It does not follow that sociology cannot be 'scientific' in the same sense as the experimental sciences of the natural world; but it can only be scientific 'in ways which are as *different* from the latter as they are specific to the nature of societies' (Bhaskar, 1994: 93; original emphasis). The objects of sociological investigation only manifest themselves in 'open systems', namely, in systems where 'invariant empirical regularities' do not obtain. This means that sociology, due to an absence of spontaneously occurring, and the impossibility of creating (i.e. through laboratory experiments), 'closures', is denied, in principle, decisive test situations for its theories. This in turn means that the criteria for the rational confirmation and rejection of theories in sociology cannot be *predictive*, and so must be *exclusively explanatory* (Bhaskar, 1989a: 83).

Adapting Bhaskar's Kantian transcendentalist mode of reasoning, it can be attested that, given the patterned findings of positivistic research, there *must* exist *real class relations* determined by the ownership/control of the means of production. The neo-Marxist theorizing of class relations developed by Clement and Myles (1997) is helpful at this point. They draw on the work of Carchedi (1977) to (re-)emphasize that classes are formed at the point of production and reproduced throughout social life. Central to class formation are the 'criteria of real economic ownership of the means of production and the appropriation of surplus value and/or value through control and surveillance of the labour of others' (referred to by Carchedi as the 'global function of capital'). The exercise of control and surveillance in relation to the process of labour is distinct from the accomplishment of 'co-ordination and unity', which is part of 'creating surplus value/labour' (referred to by Carchedi as the 'global function of the collective worker') (Clement and Myles, 1997: 12). The typology of classes yielded by this analysis – involving a *capitalist-executive class*, a *new middle class*, an *old middle class* and a *working class* – is as follows.

Clement and Myles' typologies of classes are:

1 *capitalist-executive*: those who have specific economic powers of real economic ownership, the power to direct production to specific purposes and to dispose of its products (i.e. command over 'strategic decision making');

2 *new middle class*: those who exercise 'control and surveillance' as an extension of real economic ownership (i.e. command over 'tactical decision making' about administrative processes affecting others or control/surveillance over the labour power of other employees);

3 *old middle class*: those who own their own means of realizing their labour, but work outside the dominant relations of production;

4 *working class*: those who have no command over the means of production, the labour power of others, or their own means of realizing their own labour.

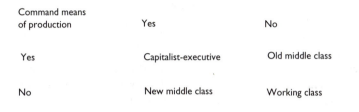

Command labour power of others

Command means of production	Yes	No
Yes	Capitalist-executive	Old middle class
No	New middle class	Working class

Figure 5.1   Class relations in Clement and Myles
Source: Adapted from Clement and Myles (1997)

The 'primary' relationship, the authors stress, is between the capitalist-executive class and the working class; but Figure 5.1 summarizes the relations between all four classes.

Having sketched, if not elaborated on or defended (see Scambler and Higgs, 1999), both an ontology (anchored in the critical realism of Bhaskar) and a non-positivistic, neo-Marxist and 'strongly relational' (Crompton, 1998) theorization of class relations (using the research of Clement and Myles), it is now time to turn to the relevant writings of Habermas. It will be maintained that his system/lifeworld dichotomy and notions of excessive system rationalization and lifeworld colonization provide a suitable framework within which to locate a theory of class relations, but also that he has permitted his (still neo-Marxist) theorization of class to atrophy somewhat and to become prematurely marginal to a proper understanding of the nature of change in high modernity.

System, lifeworld and class

Not long ago Habermas (1992: 469) described himself as 'the last Marxist', referring to a Marxian tradition 'which I've fiercely decided to defend as a still-meaningful enterprise' (1992: 465). But it is, as Sitton (1996:198) observes, a 'chastened Marxism'. Certainly Habermas has long distanced himself from what he regards as Marx's moments of 'Hegelian-inspired theology and anthropology', according to which humans are seen exclusively as producers, societies as totalities and history as progress (Love, 1995: 51). Fortunately, the often abstruse intricacies of his protracted, philosophical attempt to reconstruct a Marxian historical materialism beyond the philosophy of consciousness need not concern us here (see Rockmore, 1989); in fact, only those elements of his reconstruction that bear on class relations require comment.

It was emphasized in Chapter 1 that Habermas has consistently argued that Marx focused too much on the concept of 'work' and neglected 'interaction'; as a result he omitted to develop any prototype for Habermas' own theory of communicative action. Habermas (1984, 1987) has of course gone on to propound a theory which, in essence, allows him to distinguish between the system – comprising the economy (which generates money) and the state (which generates power), and which is characterized by strategic action (or action oriented to success) – and the lifeworld – comprising the private sphere (which generates commitment) and the public sphere (which generates influence), and which is characterized by communicative action (or action oriented to understanding). He maintains that social differentiation has led to an uncoupling of system and lifeworld, and to an excessive rationalization of the former at the cost of a colonization of the latter.

How, within this system/lifeworld framework, does Habermas analyse the capitalist economy as a subsystem in general, and class relations in particular, and how and to what extent does he depart from Marx in doing so? In venturing an answer it is convenient to start with his invocation of Marx's concept of 'real abstraction'. But Habermas' concept of real abstraction differs from that of Marx: specifically, he rejects the labour theory of value. 'Instead, Habermas uses the concept as a framework for analysing how meaningful, purposive *actions* in the lifeworld of social groups are utilized – "behind their backs" or "over their heads" – as *performances* that maintain the *functioning* of the social system as a whole' (Sitton, 1998: 66; Habermas, 1996; original emphasis).

Habermas argues that the capitalist economy must be seen as more than an arena within which labour is subordinated and exploited (i.e. in terms of classes). Marx did not distinguish between the level of system differentiation attained in modernity and the class-specific forms in which it has been institutionalized. 'Marx is convinced a priori', Habermas (1987: 339) contends, 'that in capital he has before him *nothing more* than the mystified form of a class relation. This interpretation excludes from the start the question of whether the systematic interconnection of the capitalist economy and the modern state administration do not also represent a higher and evolutionary advantageous level of integration by comparison to traditional societies' (original emphasis). For Habermas, the emergence of the discrete media-steered subsystems of the economy and state not only increases material reproduction, but also reduces the burden of processes of communication of a de-traditionalized lifeworld. The institutionalization of 'delinguistified' media such as money and power 'simplifies' social interaction in many spheres of life by reducing the conditions necessary for coordinating action. Thus prices, representing the medium of money, can transmit information that automatically coordinates the interactions of strategically acting individuals or businesses.

Habermas argues that the economic subsystem is constituted by formal law. Within it individuals are free to act strategically in accordance with legal definitions which exclude other normative considerations: the law marks off domains of 'norm-free sociality'. The economic subsystem procures the performances required for its functioning via the legal institution of the labour contract. Labour has to be 'monetarized' because the economic subsystem, *qua* subsystem – and there is more than a hint here of the systems theory of Luhmann (1982, 1995; Scambler, 1998) – 'can relate to its environment only via its own medium', money (Habermas, 1987: 292). This monetarization of labour permits the functioning of the subsystem, which delivers goods and services to be exchanged for monetary demand.

Habermas (1987) recognizes the economy is 'crisis-ridden' or subject to 'disequlibria'. Disequilibria are to be expected in a subsystem adapting to changing environments. In a capitalist economy these disequilibria are handled by another subsystem, the state; that is, by a bureaucratized administration steered by the medium of power.

Why have there been excesses of system rationalization and increasing lifeworld colonization? Why, put differently, have the subsystems of economy and state pushed beyond what is strictly necessary for the institutionalization of money and power? Like Offe, Habermas (1987) maintains that the welfare state emerged to fill in the functional gaps of the capitalist economy caused by the economic disequilibria of 'crisis-ridden growth', such as business cycles and paucity of infrastructural investment. The welfare state also occurred because of the potential for class struggle over distribution. This potential is blocked by a variety of corporatist devices resulting in wage scales set through bargaining mediated by the state, and by the direct state provision of use-values like health care. In this way 'the social antagonism bred by private disposition over the means of producing social wealth increasingly loses its structure-forming power for the lifeworld of social groups, although it does remain constitutive for the structure of the economic system' (Habermas, 1987: 348). With the steady rise in living standards, plus other state-sponsored protections of private life from system imperatives, 'conflicts over distribution also lose their explosive power' (Habermas, 1987: 349–50).

The rising standard of living and protective policies of the welfare state reduce the salience of the role of employee and enhance that of consumer. In this way, in Sitton's (1996: 173) phrase, 'class structuration in the lifeworld is obliterated'. McCarthy (1984: xix) refers here to 'the disappearance of the proletariat into the pores of consumer society'. The welfare state also transforms citizens into clients. The subsystem of the state requires legitimation, which it attains in the form of mass loyalty by providing use-values and other services that are not forthcoming from an economic subsystem that operates through exchange values. The state, to cite Sitton (1996: 173–4), 'thereby transforms citizens into clients responding to legally anchored power. Habermas even refers to this clientization of citizens as the "model case" of "colonization". This is Habermas' version of the "welfare state compromise" that has been maintained since the end of the Second World War in advanced capitalist countries.'

Habermas argues that the continued effectiveness of the welfare state compromise remains dependent on the growth of both market and welfare state. This growth results in the expansion and increasing density of the 'monetary-bureaucratic complex'. This happens where 'socially integrated contexts of life are redefined around the roles of consumer and client and assimilated to systematically integrated domains of action' (Habermas, 1987: 351). Further colonization of this sort is possible and resistance weak because the lifeworld has been de-traditionalized, its rationality potentials are 'encapsulated' in expert cultures, and it lacks the cultural resources, mobilized by an intact public sphere, to halt the intrusions of media-steering. As a consequence, 'phenomena of alienation and the unsettling of collective identity emerge' (Habermas, 1987: 386).

Habermas continues to insist that the economic subsystem retains its primacy for social evolution; but he wants to maintain also that its problems are manifested elsewhere: 'I still explain these pathologies ("loss of meaning, anomic conditions, psychopathologies") by referring to the mechanisms driving capitalism forward, namely economic growth, but I assess them in terms of the systematically induced predominance of economic and bureaucratic, indeed of all cognitive-instrumental forms of rationality with a one-sided or "alienated" everyday communicative practice' (Habermas, 1991: 2250). 'Pathologies', then, replace social crisis.

For Habermas, the classical socialist project must be amended. The importance of media-steered subsystems for social evolution has to be accepted. Sitton (1998:71) summarizes: 'A further rationalized lifeworld – one in which culture, social order and socialization are increasingly based on a consensus achieved through reasoned discourse rather than on traditional understandings – requires an unburdening of social co-ordination that can only be actualized by maintaining areas of social interaction steered not by communicative action but by media-steered subsystems. It is only through such further rationalization that the encroachment of media-steered subsystems can be successfully resisted and the reproduction of the lifeworld secured.'

There is much in Habermas' reformulations of Marx, his theory of communicative action, system/lifeworld dichotomy and notions of selective rationalization and lifeworld colonization which helps 'situate' and 'frame' the theorization of class outlined earlier deploying the neo-Marxist arguments and analyses of Bhaskar and Clement and Myles. But there are also, it will be maintained, significant deficiencies in his approach to class.

It is appropriate to start with Scott's (1996: 2) reminder that 'while people in their everyday lives may, indeed, now be less likely to identify themselves in "class" terms, this does not mean that class relations, as objective realities, have disappeared'. While Habermas certainly cannot be said to deny class relations as objective realities, there is a sense in which he 'persistently empties the concept of class and its contents' (Sitton, 1996: 187). Arguably it is a case of – at times careless, and at times wilful – theoretical neglect, resulting in a general process of atrophy and some conspicuous lacunae. A few more substantive critical points might be made to clarify and illustrate this.

Habermas (1987) appears to arrive at an overly narrow grasp of the potential for conflict in contemporary capitalism. He understandably emphasizes the altered character of social protest, rightly tracing the origins of an array of 'new' social movements to resistance to clientalism and consumerism. But there is strong evidence from labour history to suggest that the commodification of labour is unlikely to remain unchallenged indefinitely and cannot be 'normalized' in the way that Habermas' concessions to systems theory seem to require; in other words, there may well yet be resurgence of 'old' or class-based movements.

An important aspect of Habermas' theory is of course that class conflict has been 'tamed' in present-day capitalism by an improved standard of living and the interventionist welfare state. While he explicitly acknowledges that conflicts over distribution will return in the event of an arrest in economic growth and welfare cuts, it is not altogether clear how – ironically given the current evidence of recession and welfare state 'crisis' – his (systems-influenced) theory can accommodate such a return: as Sitton (1998: 79) points out, his theory was after all intended to 'explain the discontents with a successful welfare state compromise'.

If system imperatives are to be confronted and blocked in the name of a decolonization and extended rationalization of the lifeworld, itself arguably a continuation of the Marxist project, the ways in which relations of class affect media-steering in relation to both the economy and state require to be analysed in more detail than Habermas allows. A reconstruction of the public sphere of the lifeworld may be necessary to overcome the fragmentation of consciousness – which Habermas sees as having now replaced 'false consciousness' – that obstructs an effective opposition to system imperatives; but 'if we are to do away with the "fetishism of the labour market" the instrumental dimension of connecting discourse with binding decisions must be broached' (Sitton, 1996: 198). If it is not, then, as Fraser (1992) has maintained, the public sphere will simply be overrun and rendered impotent. 'Cultural revolution has never been enough' (Sitton, 1996: 198).

A final comment here concerns the globalization of capitalism. Capitalism's system imperatives now play themselves out on a global stage. Capitalism must be analysed as transnational or as a world-system: 'it is here that the system escapes the lifeworld if anywhere' (Sitton, 1996: 199). Habermas' analysis of selective, or excessive, system rationalization and lifeworld colonization requires to be supplemented by a consideration of the historical and contemporary effects of the colonization of nations and peoples and of national lifeworld resistance to such colonization. The theme of globalization plays an important part in the next section of this chapter.

Power elite and capitalist-executive

To recap, it has been suggested so far that medical sociologists' flawed positivistic contributions to the understanding of health inequalities have been limited also by failures to adequately theorize class relations; an ontology of class relations deriving from the philosophy of Bhaskar has been proposed; a feasible neo-Marxist class schema developed by Clement and Myles, involving a capitalist-executive, new and old middle classes and a working class, has been outlined; and the theories of Habermas have been plumbed, both positively, to utilize his theory of communicative action and system/lifeworld framework, and negatively, to highlight important deficiencies in his analysis of class.

In this and the next section, building on these theoretical and conceptual preparations, the 'greedy bastards hypothesis' (GBH), namely, *that health inequalities in Britain can be reasonably interpreted as indirect (and largely unintended) consequences of the ever-adaptive behaviours of members of Britain's power elite and capitalist-executive*, will be elaborated in some detail. The intention in this and the next section is not to 'test' this complex and awkward hypothesis, which would be premature, but rather to explore the conditions and extent of its plausibility, and to reflect on how effective empirical procedures to test it might be devised. The justification for this degree of caution should become clear.

The idea of a power elite and its putative association with the capitalist-executive must first be clarified. But any sensible explication rests on an adequate understanding of the changing nature of late-twentieth-century 'disorganized' capitalism. A brief synopsis will have to suffice.

It has become commonplace for sociologists not only to document a historical progression from 'liberal' capitalism (characterized by a 'facilitative' state) to 'organized' capitalism (characterized by an 'interventionist' state), but also to record a more recent transition from organized to 'disorganized' capitalism (with states typically remaining more interventionist than facilitative) (Offe, 1985; Lash and Urry, 1987). Habermas is one of many to chart the growth of welfare state interventionism consequent upon the progression from liberal to organized capitalism, and to note that this functioned to take the sting out of conflicts of class; to supply those use-values and other services required for the reproduction of capitalist activity but which were beyond the capacity of the economy itself to provide; and increasingly, to restructure and support private capital. The disorganization of capitalist production can be dated – politically, at least – from the 1970s, from which time nation-states started to dismantle their interventionist and planning structures and to promote the 'de-regulation' of many areas of economic activity.

Scott (1986, 1997: 264–5) points out that while state expenditure during organized capitalism led to an increase in the productivity of capital, a portion of this productivity was (and is yet) required to finance current and future state expenditure, 'and unless private productivity grows along with the growth of state expenditure there will be a decline in the rate of capital accumulation ... State intervention becomes a necessary support for private capital that nevertheless poses problems for private profitability and so makes further public expenditure more difficult to finance.' The expansion of state intervention and collective provision also results in political dislocations within the state itself. To cite Habermas (1976) once more, economic 'crisis tendencies' do not vanish with welfare statism but rather become displaced into the state's own structure. States seek to accommodate their budgetary problems through regulatory policies, but in a private enterprise system there are determinate limits to state power. In the words of Scott (1997: 265), 'rather than securing an independent and autonomous policy or one that is in the "general interests" of capital, states are likely to pursue policies that reflect a balance of power among the various capitalist interests represented within their agencies. Consensual state policies, to the extent that they occur, are consequences of the dominance of particular fractions of capital within the state apparatus.'

In the stage of disorganized capitalism, born out of the 'devastation of the 1970s' (Sklair, 1998: 152), national economies have become disarticulated: in particular, economic interests have become more routinely globalized. 'Capitalist families and capitalist enterprises alike are locked into globalized circuits of capital and investment that are no longer organized around distinctively national economies' (Scott, 1997: 298; see also Eichengreen, 1996). Some have argued that as relations of class have become more global, national capitalist classes have become increasingly fragmented (e.g. Arrighi et al., 1989). Others, like Sklair (1995, 1998), have asked whether it is appropriate now to refer to a 'transnational capitalist class'.

Sklair's (1998: 136) own neo-Marxist global system theory is rooted in the notion of transnational practices, that is, 'practices that are abstracted from national class systems in that they cross state boundaries and do not necessarily originate with state agencies or actors'. He contends that the dominating forces of global capitalism are the dominating forces of the global system, adding that the building blocks of this theory – in the economic, political and culture-ideological spheres respectively – are the transnational corporations, a still-evolving transnational capitalist class, and the culture-ideology of consumerism. He divides the transnational capitalist class analytically into four principal fractions: the executives of transnational corporations, globalizing bureaucrats, globalizing politicians and professionals, and consumerist elites (merchants and media). 'My argument', writes Sklair (1998: 137), 'is that those who dominate these groups, taken together, constitute a global power elite, ruling class or inner circle in the sense that these terms have been used to characterise the class structures of specific countries' (see Domhoff, 1967; Scott, 1996; Useem, 1984).

Scott (1997: 313) thinks it premature of Sklair to put his faith in concepts like 'transnational capitalist class' and 'global power elite'. But for all his neo-Weberian caution, Scott himself, in one of the most impressive and exhaustive surveys of the empirical literature, notes, against much received wisdom, sociological as well as non-sociological, that, despite the transition from organized to disorganized capitalism, propertied families remain a potent economic and political force; these families, he adds, 'are far from having their privileges usurped by upwardly mobile career managers'. And his closing sentences read: 'the emergence of impersonal possession has resulted merely in a managerial reorganization of the propertied class. Wealthy families have diversified their income-earning assets, and many now participate in strategic control on the basis of mechanisms other than direct inheritance of a place in the family firm. In the stage of disorganized capitalism, however, the members of this class have become involved in the more extensive transnational economic practices that are disarticulating their national economies. National capitalist classes have themselves become more fragmented and "disorganized", and their futures may – though this is, as yet, unclear – involve the formation of a global capitalist class.'

Towards the conclusion of his lucid and witty historical depiction of the 'wealth and poverty of nations', Landes (1998: 520) notes that 'men of money can buy men of power', adding that contemporary presidents and prime ministers 'act as traveling salesmen and judge their success by deals closed and contracts signed'. It has been argued in similar vein elsewhere that Britain has an identifiable power elite which is infused and informed by its capitalist-executive (Higgs and Scambler, 1998; Scambler and Higgs, 1999). This statement can now be elaborated.

If all societies with a state necessarily have a state or political elite, they may not all have a power elite. Scott's (1991: 118–19) way of making this distinction is to claim that 'the occupants of positions of authority within the state elite compromise a power elite only where they are recruited from a power bloc'; and he defines a power bloc as 'an alignment of social groups having some similarity in social background and experience and which is able to monopolise positions of authority within the state elite over a sustained period'. A power bloc too must attain 'consciousness', 'coherence' and 'conspiracy' (or coordination); that is, it must evolve some awareness of common interests and concerns, some degree of solidarity and cohesion, and its leading representatives must be capable of coordinated policies of action to further the bloc's interests (Scott, 1991: 122). Scott, one of the most diligent comparative researchers in this area, offers convincing evidence for the existence of a power bloc and a power elite in Britain.

In the same text Scott maintains further that the British state also operates in the interests of a particular – that is, its capitalist – class; state power in Britain, in other words, has a class character. Adopting Therborn's (1978: 144) phrasing, state power can be said to have a class character when what is accomplished through the state apparatus 'positively acts upon the (re-)production of the mode of production, of which the class in question is the dominant bearer'. A state operates in the interests of a capitalist class, Scott (1991: 139) claims, 'when its activities reinforce the conditions for the reproduction of that class and it fails to act in ways which undermine these conditions'. Scott's (1991: 151) response to the fundamental question he sets out to answer – 'Who rules Britain?' – is unequivocal: 'Britain is ruled by a capitalist class whose economic dominance is sustained by the operations of the state and whose members are disproportionately represented in the power elite which rules the state apparatus.' According to his preferred terminology, Britain has a 'ruling class'.

Scott (1991: 89–90) sees the capitalist class as increasingly dependent on a system of impersonal capital resulting from the expansion of institutional property holdings: it comprises entrepreneurial capitalists, 'passive' rentiers and executive capitalists, and has an 'inner circle' of finance capitalists with two or more directorships in very large enterprises in the system of impersonal capital. Its members have acquired a new global mobility. Bauman (1998: 9) describes them appositely as 'absentee landlords, mark II'. Scott estimates the size of this class at 0.1 per cent of the adult population, some 43,500 individuals.

It would of course be naïve and erroneous to assume either that the power elite invariably does the bidding of the leading representatives of the capitalist-executive (returning here to the label and definition of Clement and Myles), or that members of the capitalist-executive routinely think and act as one. For all his recognition of the pre-potent class-oriented functions of the state in capitalist societies, and of the growing density and colonizing ways of the 'monetary-bureaucratic complex', Habermas' (1976, 1987) analysis of the complex interchanges between the state and the private and public spheres of the lifeworld makes it clear that a state's power elite cannot *simply* and *always* respond to a capitalist-executive. What is required, in fact, is that the activities of the apparatus of the state 'do not undermine the existing relations of production and continue, in the long term, to reinforce them' (Scott, 1991: 140).

That the capitalist-executive, or for that matter its leading personnel, or members of the power bloc or even the power elite, rarely attain total unanimity or speak with a single voice is also apparent (although, as Scott insists of members of the power bloc, they must be able to act with consciousness, coherence and with a capacity for conspiracy/coordination *when it matters*). This lack of unanimity, as Sklair (1998) is quick to concede, is perhaps especially true in the stage of disorganized, or global, capitalism, with the transfer of the large enterprises that act as the 'visible hands' of capital, together with the 'invisible handshakes' through which these enterprises influence each other, to the international level (Scott, 1997: 256). Key British economic and political divisions on future scenarios for the European Union testify to the realities of dissensus. But recognition of the existence of real divisions of opinion and fractionalization around issues among elites should not of course be confused with the rejection of neo-Marxist (and other equivalent) perspectives in favour of more superficial 'pluralist' alternatives.

The undoubted, if partial, globalization of Britain's power elite, as well as the more robust or advanced globalization of those elements of its capitalist-executive that shape its policy and practices, have as yet been more often acknowledged than studied, at least sociologically (see Held *et al.*, 1999). But it is important to note that awareness of these globalizing processes has helped promote a series of assumptions concerning the dissipation or fragmentation of class consciousness (which are possibly justified, albeit with qualification (Marshall *et al.*, 1988)) and the declining significance of class relations (which are not). Once the point of analysis shifts from the nation-state to the world-system, the proposition that relations of class have lost their salience seems a good deal less seductive (see Chase-Dunn, 1989).

Remaining at the global level, during his discussion and advocacy of the concept of a transnational capitalist class, Sklair (1998: 140) makes a key point, namely, that 'the culture-ideology of consumerism is the fundamental value system that keeps the system intact'. And later, in more detail: 'the point of the concept of culture-ideology of consumerism is precisely that, under capitalism, the masses can not be relied upon to keep buying when they have neither spare cash nor access to credit, and, less obviously, even when they do have spare cash and access to credit'. 'The modern world-system', Wallerstein (1998: 10) writes, 'was, and is, a capitalist system, that is, a system that operates on the primacy of the endless accumulation of capital via the eventual commodification of everything.' The creation of a culture-ideology of consumerism, therefore, is bound up with the self-imposed necessity that capitalism must be ever-expanding on a global scale. 'This expansion crucially depends on selling more and more goods and services to people whose basic needs (a somewhat ideological term) have already been comfortably met, as well as to those whose basic needs have not been met' (Sklair, 1998: 148–9).

Relations of class are critical for grasping the ideological role of consumerism (as they are for a proper appreciation of the state's substitution of clients for citizens). It is astonishing how frequently those concerned to record a switch from productivism under organized capitalism to consumerism under disorganized capitalism have neglected or even overlooked these ideological properties. The temptation to minimize the 'continuities' of recent capitalism might be less if the adjective 'reorganized' was substituted for 'disorganized' in relation to its contemporary stage (Ashley, 1997).

A final point concerns the putative fragility of today's global, disorganized – or reorganized – capitalism (and the account here requires only a cautious commitment to what Held and colleagues (1999) refer to as a 'transformationalist' view of globalization, midway, say, between the stances of Scott and Sklair). It would of course be premature to regard capitalism itself as fragile. Nor is it that the power elite and capitalist-executive are less obdurately and subtly adaptive now than was the case during either liberal or organized capitalism. It is rather that since the mid-1980s novel forms of instability have come apace to threaten the world's money, debt, equity and derivative markets, and not only in the minds of speculators like Soros (1998) (see, for example, Warburton, 1999). There is real uncertainty, even in the short term.

To summarize at the close of this section, it has been maintained that there is sound empirical evidence favouring the existence of a 'weakly globalized' power elite at the core of the subsystem of the state in Britain, which owes a binding *de facto* allegiance, primarily if not exclusively, since it must be responsive too to the private and public spheres of the lifeworld, to a 'strongly globalized' capitalist-executive in the economic subsystem. In this sense, close to Scott's, there is a ruling capitalist class in Britain. This class is the principal source for the diffusion of strategic action, for selective rationalization, and for the colonization of the lifeworld.

Neither the power elite nor the capitalist-executive are without fractions and dissensus, although there is almost invariably a unanimity of purpose and action where and when it matters, that is, around issues perceived of as important for the relations of production in the longer term. Class relations, then, remain of central significance for attempts, either within nation-states or globally, to account for phenomena like order, conflict and change. They are no less central for our understanding of the ideological properties not only of consumerism but also of clientalism. While Habermas may have been ill-advised to have paid so little attention to relations of class in his writings in the 1990s, and his system/lifeworld framework arguably requires further refinement, both to allow for the continuing structural, political and ideological significance of class relations and to accommodate processes of globalization, it is not apparent that these 'refinements' cannot be made without jeopardizing his theory of communicative action (now extended to a discourse ethics).

What has been called here the fragility of disorganized capitalism has also not been adequately treated by Habermas, chiefly perhaps because he has been busy with other matters, notably philosophical aspects of constitutional law and democratic practice. While it would be foolish to regard capitalism as 'in crisis', it would be no less so, given the present degrees of instability and unpredictability in financial markets, to rule out a resurgence – at local, regional, national, or even transnational levels – of more overt forms of class disputation, conflict and activity, and possibly, of 'old' labour movements. While the emphasis of Habermas and of many other European theorists has (in many ways, understandably) switched from old to 'new' social movements as agents of change, it would be a mistake to be too dismissive of the former and too hopeful for the latter; like many of his colleagues, Habermas is in fact too dismissive of the former, if not too hopeful for the latter (for more discussion of these issues, see Chapter 9).

Class, power and health inequalities

It is not difficult to construct a *prima facie* case for the hypothesis that health inequalities in capitalist nations like Britain might be interpreted as indirect (and largely unintended) consequences of the single-minded but adaptive behaviours of members of its power elite and capitalist-executive, each of these being subject to novel processes of globalization (Higgs and Scambler, 1998; Scambler and Higgs, 1999). That this is so is due in no small part to the enduring contradictions of capitalism. Habermas' (1976) argument in *Legitimation Crisis* still applies, albeit with a new global edge: independently of the rate of a nation's economic growth and of the comprehensiveness of its welfare state, the fundamental contradiction between the social process of production and the private appropriation and use of the product remains. The priorities of the 'system' are not based on generalizable interests, but on the private goals of profit maximization.

In other words, the kinds of disparities of wealth and income found in Britain (see Dean and Melrose, 1999) – and in other capitalist societies (see Atkinson, 1998) – are to be expected, since they are necessary concomitants of the *de facto* realization of system – or, more precisely, economic subsystem – priorities. Moreover, because they largely determine differential material standards of living (and less conspicuously much else that relates to material standard of living, from housing tenure and quality, local amenities and car ownership to a vast array of well-documented cognitions and risk behaviours for health), these disparities also serve causally to underpin the production and reproduction of health inequalities and the state's consistent failure to intervene to ameliorate them.

The essential point to emphasize here is that it is class relations, and in particular the behaviours of members of the power elite as well as of the capitalist-executive, which are *above all else* defined by those relations, that effectively underwrite the enduring character of health inequalities. That this is rarely the intention behind their decision and policies, which are driven *above all else* by the accumulation of capital over the longer term, might seem obvious, but perhaps requires some elaboration.

In the remainder of this section further brief comments are offered on four (sets of) issues arising from the discussion so far: (1) the distinction, utilized within the GBH, between the intended and unintended consequences of the behaviours of members of the power elite and capitalist-executive; (2) the range of 'levels' of causal influence and penetration of class relations (as theorized here) germane to the production, reproduction and enduring nature of health inequalities; (3) some implications of the theorization of class relations for other, complementary or alternative, sources of health inequalities, especially gender and ethnicity; and (4) some thoughts on a viable future research agenda for medical sociologists.

Intended and unintended consequences of the behaviours of members of the power elite/capitalist-executive

When considering the claim that continuing health inequalities might be interpreted as 'indirect (and largely unintended) consequences' of the single-minded but adaptive behaviours of members of Britain's power elite and capitalist-executive, at least three pertinent dimensions or axes warrant attention, namely, *instrumentality*, *contextuality* and *reflexivity*.

First, it should perhaps be reiterated that the behaviours of members of the power elite, critically informed by core members of the capitalist-executive, are defined by their *instrumentality* (in Habermas' terms, they are strategic not communicative, operating, respectively, through the steering-media of power and money). They are directed at the accumulation of capital over the longer term, other considerations being at once secondary and salient only under effective pressure either from re-invigorated labour movements or from the mobilizing activities of new social movements in the public sphere of the lifeworld. There is little evidence or prospect of such telling pressure in contemporary Britain.

Second, it is congruent with the hypothesis commended here to accept that *in any given context* instances of the behaviours of representatives of the power elite and capitalist-executive might promote, arrest or inhibit health inequalities; and the outcome might vary also according to the time-frame adopted. Although the GBH maintains that health inequalities can be interpreted as (largely unintended) consequences of these behaviours, it remains the case that in 'exceptional' contexts these behaviours might serve to stall, mitigate against or reduce health inequalities. The recent bargaining over the future of Rover production affords a possible example, and with a strong globalizing theme. Given the well-documented association between (even the threat of) job loss and impoverished health, both for those involved and for their partners and children (see Smith, 1987; Bartley, 1994), the 'deal' apparently struck (at the time of writing) between Munich-based Joachim Milberg of BMW and Industry Secretary Stephen Byers to resuscitate Rover car production at the Longbridge plant, thereby preserving some 10,000 jobs at the plant and at least as many jobs outside it, might, *if it sticks* (and one must be sceptical), prevent some further deepening of health inequalities in the West Midlands through the next decade (Bannister and White, 1999).

Third, those behaviours that serve to extend, or far more exceptionally to arrest or counter, health inequalities may be prosecuted either with or without *reflexivity*, that is, with or without awareness of their probable health implications. An additional refinement of the hypothesis might be that the behaviours are (increasingly) more likely to be reflexive – yet 'cynical', in Bourdieu's sense (quoted in Bauman, 1999: 2) – than non-reflexive, even among core members of the capitalist-executive; but that, as Bauman (1998: 10) elsewhere argues, one consequence of globalization – and potential, although presently quite remote, source of a crisis of legitimacy for the state – is a diminution of a sense of responsibility or 'duty' on the part of capitalist decision-makers: 'the costs of coping with the consequences need not be now counted in the calculation of the "effectiveness of investment" ' (see also Bauman, 1998a).

Thus the pivotal behaviours of key personnel in the weakly globalized power elite and strongly globalized capitalist-executive in Britain, which are paradigmatically instrumental and indicative of growing reflexivity, are typically, that is, in most contexts, conducive to the production and reproduction of health inequalities. Moreover, these inequalities, rooted as they are in the contradictions of capitalism itself, cannot be significantly ameliorated in the continuing absence of (effectively decolonizing) resistance from either old or new social movements.

Class relations, levels of causality and health inequalities

The most distinctive aspect of the theorization of class epitomized here, beyond its explicit and substantive neo-Marxist properties, is probably its ontological basis in Bhaskar's critical realist philosophy. The objects of sociological enquiry, it has been maintained, are both real and necessarily 'theoretical' (in that they are necessarily unperceivable); they cannot be studied – and do not exist – independently of their effects. Relations of class fall into this category. It has been suggested too, again adopting Bhaskar's transcendentalist reasoning, that, given the consistent patterning of positivist data on health (and other) inequalities, there *must* exist *real relations of class* turning on the *ownership/control of the means of production*. But this is a starting point for empirical research, not its conclusion.

Positivism sticks with the perceivable. Under-theorized operationalizations of (occupational) class in readiness for abstruse forms of multivariate analysis, reducing class to the status of other 'variables' like height, public examination results or car ownership, occur in anticipation of viable inferences to the causal power of class on the basis of degrees of statistical association. Even the more feasible schema of Popperian (neo-positivist) 'falsificationism' remains untapped (Popper, 1963, 1972). If it is questionable whether this flawed set of procedures should have any residual appeal for epidemiologists (Krieger, 1994), it should long have been beyond the pale for medical sociologists. Sociologists are rather required to study theoretical – or unperceivable – objects, albeit through their effects in open systems. Relations of class typically take effect or 'bite' indirectly and 'behind people's back'.

When Habermas (1987: 117) claims that the subsystems of the economy and state, operating through their steering-media of money and power, 'stabilise nonintended interconnections of actions by way of functionally intermeshing "action consequences"', carrying the implication that the 'functional significance of actions is not identical to action orientations' (Sitton, 1998: 75), he is surely right; but what he neglects is the role of class relations in general, and of the power elite informed and harried by the capitalist-executive in particular, in the uncoupling of system and lifeworld, in selective rationalization, and in the genesis, institutional consolidation and continued colonizing force of the subsystems of economy and state. He has, it seems, allowed class to go missing of late.

What then of the causal contribution of class relations to enduring health inequalities? Medical sociologists have been exhorted elsewhere to focus on both the nature and extent of the embeddedness of – it is frequently claimed, causally-linked chains or webs of – *risk factors* for health in class relations (Scambler and Higgs, 1999). Making her own case against positivist methods, but this time as deployed by epidemiologists, not least around the image of a 'web of causation', Krieger aptly poses the question: 'Has anyone seen the spider?' Towards the end of her discussion she writes: 'To forge a better theory, it may still be worthwhile to search for the "spider". Whether there is one spider or many', she adds, 'can be determined only if this task is pursued' (Krieger, 1994: 899). It is surely a compulsory task for sociologists in this area. The GBH, articulated in terms of the British power elite/capitalist-executive, postulates class as – at a parsimonious minimum – the most impressive and diligent spider currently at work.

But just how influential a spider is class? It is of heuristic value at this point to refer to the Whitehead/Dhalgren 'model', which distinguishes five 'levels' or 'modes of explanation' in relation to health inequalities (Dhalgren and Whitehead, 1991; for a critical exposition, see Popay *et al.*, 1998). At the first level or mode of explanation are the biological givens of sex and age, as well as those qualities inherited from biological parents. These factors are beyond individuals' control, and include those environmental forces that shaped their parents' health at the time they were conceived, and even their grandparents' health at the time of their parents' conceptions (see Barker, 1991).

At the second level are 'lifestyle factors', over which individuals are thought by most to have some degree of control. These include smoking, alcohol consumption, eating patterns and the taking of exercise. Studies of 'risk factor epidemiology', as it is sometimes termed, have proved irresistible to many medical sociologists (Scambler and Higgs, 1999; Levinson, 1998). Syme (1996: 23), an epidemiologist, has referred to it somewhat scathingly as 'clinical medicine in large groups'.

Levels three and four – 'social and community influences' and 'living and working conditions' respectively – for all that they might be said to 'envelop' lifestyle factors and are thereby more appealing to Syme, are also interpreted individualistically in the Whitehead/Dhalgren model and by most researchers (Popay *et al.*, 1998). The Whitehall studies are (epidemiological) exemplars of such research, having moved beyond an exclusive engagement at level two to encompass levels three and, especially, four (Marmot *et al.*, 1978, 1991).

The fifth level or mode of explanation represents 'the material aspects of the context within which individual and population health is located – aspects which are largely determined by national and international forces' (Popay *et al.*, 1998: 63). Low income, poor housing and unemployment are pertinent examples here, all of which have been linked to health inequalities by a substantial body of research.

It now seems apparent that if relations of class, as defined in this chapter, (still) have salience for health inequalities in today's disorganized or reorganized capitalism, their impact is most likely to be felt at level five, causally determining and sustaining phenomena like income inequality. A case can be made, however, that they retain a role at *all* levels in the genesis and perpetuation of those conditions – including over the course of time those at the first level – conducive to the production and reproduction of health inequalities. Of prime importance in this context are those 'mechanisms' – across the economic, political and cultural-ideological spheres – functionally required by the 'logic' of the economic subsystem and substantially underwritten by the power elite and capitalist-executive, which in turn render secure an important subset of those conditions (at each level in the Whitehead/Dhalgren model) conducive to health inequalities. Class relations, to risk a further analogy, are the likely 'key' that 'locks' such mechanisms (and the key presently remains in the safe-keeping of the power elite/capitalist-executive).

Other sources of health inequalities

The theorization of class relations outlined here is undeniably provisional, and not merely in the obvious sense that all theories of both social and natural phenomena necessarily remain fallible and open to future revision. The principal lacuna is probably the failure to give sufficient attention to the effects of what Bauman (1999: 40), following Hobsbawm, calls the 'uneven and unsynchronized' processes of globalization on class relations in nation-states like Britain. In fact few medical sociologists have sound records for analyses beyond the territorial boundaries of their own states (for an exception in relation not only to class but also to gender, see Doyal, 1979, 1995).

Apart from class relations, relations of gender and ethnicity are foremost among numerous 'rival' candidates in accounting for health inequalities. Neither can be reduced to class. Nor, as has frequently occurred in the positivist research on health inequalities, should they (only) be analysed independently of class (MacIntyre and Hunt, 1997; Nazroo, 1998). Picking up on the discussion above, it is certainly not enough either to state that women and members of ethnic minority groups are under-represented in the power elite and in the decisive echelons of the capitalist-executive, although, importantly, they continue to be so. Clement and Myles (1997: 140) point the way here, and are surely right to insist, with reference to gender, that 'class relations are not just class relations', and to maintain that 'relations of power and authority in the modern workplace exist not only to regulate relations between capital and labour but also to reproduce a particular way of organising relations between men and women. The class structures of the developed capitalist economies are also neo-patriarchal structures, a system of rule by senior males that by and large excludes women from exercising power over men.' Lacking data, the authors leave open the question as to whether the process generating a neo-patriarchal pattern of production relations 'is exclusively a class, not a gender, process', but conjecture that this is unlikely.

The same might be said of ethnicity as of gender. In his consideration of extant research on ethnicity and health inequalities, Nazroo (1998: 167) notes too that one by-product of the highly focused preoccupation with the empirical delineation of 'pathways' – at their most ambitious, from levels five to one in the Whitehead/Dhalgren model – is that 'the root cause, wider social inequalities, becomes obscured from view'. Commending the arguments of Williams and associates (1994) in the USA, he concludes by asserting that 'we need to remember that we are concerned with (ethnic) inequalities in health because they are a component and a consequence of an inequitable capitalist society, and it is this that needs to be directly addressed'.

There is a need, then, not only for an adequate theorization of relations of class in the investigation of health inequalities, but also for adequate theorizations of, for example, gender and ethnic relations, and of the interfaces between class, gender and ethnic relations as these pertain to health inequalities.

Future research

The argument has been advanced elsewhere (Scambler and Higgs, 1999), and was outlined earlier, that a credible, explicitly sociological and neo-Marxist theorization of the *reality* of class relations might be grounded in the philosophical theses of Bhaskar. Such a theorization, it will be recalled, carries the implication that sociology is fundamentally explanatory and committed to the study of such ('beneath the surface') objects as relations of class – and of gender and ethnicity – which are however only accessible through their *effects* ('on the surface') in ineluctably 'open systems'. The methodological ramifications are stark and uncomfortable. The currently dominant, albeit untenable, positivist research programme on health inequalities remains predictive – or rather views explanation and prediction as two sides of the same coin – and committed to the study of variables ('on the surface') in contexts too readily defined as quasi-experimental 'closures'. Life for any researcher adopting a post-positivist agenda of the kind indicated in this chapter is a good deal more complex.

This complexity can be illustrated by reference to the need for three related types of innovation: *theoretical, conceptual* and *methodological*. The present chapter's focus on the salience of the power elite and capitalist-executive for health inequalities in Britain is an example of theoretical innovation in the sense intended, not because it is intrinsically novel – much of it has antecedents stretching back to the 1960s, even to the 1860s – but because it purports to put the medical *sociological* investigation of health inequalities (back) on a testable theoretical footing. And the GBH is of course suggestive of many other hypotheses. To pick a single unexplored example, consider the work of Elias (1991; and see van Krieken, 1998) and his concept of 'habitus', a word he employed long before Bourdieu. Habitus refers to 'second nature' or 'embodied social learning'. 'The fortunes of a nation over the centuries', he suggests in his volume *The Germans* (Elias, 1996: 19), 'become sedimented into the habitus of its individual members.' It would surely repay those medical sociologists in pursuit of a sociological explanation of health inequalities to investigate the nature and extent of the congruity between the – 'possibly calibrated or differentiated' – British habitus and people's passivity in the face of remarkably enduring health inequalities? This is not just a matter, of course, of enquiring into lay conceptions of the 'reasons for health inequalities' (Blaxter, 1997).

The urgent requirement for conceptual innovation is axiomatic. If, following Bhaskar, sociology's objects of study are 'networks of relations', like class, which are necessarily theoretical – that is, they cannot be empirically identified, nor yet exist, independently of their effects – then there is a critical and inescapable challenge to devise new modes of conceptualization for such relations – concerning, for example, *both* (increasingly globalized) relations of class, gender and ethnicity *and* the ways in which these interact – which are pertinent to the development of substantive, testable sociological theories.

Methodologically, there is a need to move beyond positivism, not, again, because *nothing* can be gleaned from positivist research, but because it is philosophically irredeemable and its sociological return unacceptably frugal. The presently ubiquitous, if largely unspoken, positivist rationale, which underpins not only the (futile) quantitative pursuit of invariant empirical regularities, but also – and somewhat counter-intuitively – much qualitative research, requires exorcism. Operating 'on the surface', positivist quantitative and qualitative studies alike typically betray a misjudgement of the potential for theory generation and testing.

Much of the complexity inherent in any convincing interrogation of the neo-Marxist perspective on class and health inequalities promoted here, or, more specifically, of the GBH, is due then to the fact that the proper objects of sociological research only manifest themselves in open systems, that is, in systems where, most conspicuously, invariant empirical regularities are not to be found. This suggests the need for a subtle triangulation of methods

(Denzin, 1989), with less emphasis than is the case in the current positivist research programme on quantitative studies and more on calculatingly post-positivist qualitative ones.

Qualitative studies consistent with this criterion might take a number of different forms, many of them well established. *Documentary analysis*, not least of the published accounts and audits of national and transnational corporations and of the conduct of government business, might pay dividends for medical sociologists interested in the social genesis of health inequalities. Detailed *life histories* afford another technique. But as the account above suggests, if life histories are to offer illumination of the causal origins of health inequalities in relations of class – as well as of gender, ethnicity and so on – then they might more usefully address the biographies of members of the power elite/capitalist-executive than those of representatives of chronically unemployed and/or sick manual workers.

Case studies complemented by 'analytic induction' also commend themselves (see Becker, 1998: 194–212). However, even small series of case studies, applying analytic induction and something of C. Wright Mills' (1959) 'sociological imagination', should not be confined to the socially disadvantaged and/or sick, but used as well, and perhaps more urgently, with the rich and powerful. Finally, mention might be made of *theoretical sampling* allied to *grounded theory*, which has assumed a variety of promising (rival) forms since it was first 'discovered' in the mid-1960s (Glaser and Strauss, 1967; Strauss and Corbin, 1990; Glaser, 1992).

What underlies this austere and rather *ad hoc* set of recom-mended qualitative approaches is a recognition that fully sociological research on class and health inequalities is likely to remain modestly, if importantly, *exploratory* for the foreseeable future. Indeed, an (arguably overdue) appreciation of the nature of the true, unperceivable, theoretical objects of sociological research, of the discipline's necessarily explanatory rather than predictive brief, and of the properties of open systems, brings with it an obligation to take more seriously than medical sociolo-gists focused on health inequalities have done hitherto the requirement for both theoretical, and – perhaps especially – conceptual, innovation. There is a need to re-think the *how* as well as the *why* in relation to the sociological investigation of health inequalities.

Conclusion

The principal objective in this chapter has been to spell out, elaborate upon and render feasible a single conjecture, albeit in the light of the dominant positivist research programme on health inequalities an audacious and far-reaching one, which also calls for novel and creative modes of testing. This was that health inequalities can plausibly be interpreted as the indirect (and largely unintended) consequences of the behaviours of members of the power elite informed by the capitalist-executive.

After briefly defining the need for a post-positivist stance in relation to research on class and health inequalities in medical sociology, the work of, first, Bhaskar and, second, Clement and Myles, was used to propose a realist, neo-Marxist and explicitly sociological orientation both to sociological objects like relations of class and to future investigations of health inequalities. The theoretical contributions of Habermas on the changing nature of contemporary capitalist society were then discussed, and it was argued that, for all the virtues of his evolving system/lifeworld framework and ideas of selective rationalization and lifeworld colonization, he has ceased to take class sufficiently seriously and allowed the notion to atrophy. The concepts of the power elite and capitalist-executive were then explicated in some depth prior to returning to issues around the enduring nature of health inequalities.

One general ramification of the preceding discussion for 'future research' is perhaps worth reiterating. The positivist methods still adopted by many medical sociologists tackling health inequalities, especially but not exclusively in the quantitative vein, have unsurprisingly had a limited yield. What is required in their place, it has been contended, is a critical and post-positivist mix of theoretical, conceptual and methodological innovations. But it must be acknowledged too that the kind of sociological hypothesis presented here does not admit of the kind of decisive testing (wrongly) assumed to be available by and to those with positivist inclinations.

References

Adonis, A. and Pollard, S. (1997) *A Class Act: The Myth of Britain's Classless Society*. London: Hamish Hamilton.
Arrighi, G., Hopkins, T. and Wallerstein, E. (1989) *Antisystematic Movements*. London: Verso.

Ashley, D. (1997) *History without a Subject: The Postmodern Condition*. Oxford: Westview Press.

Atkinson, A. (1998) *Poverty in Europe*. Oxford: Blackwell.

Bannister, N. and White, M. (1999) 'Longbridge: safe at last'. *Finance Guardian*, Thursday, 1 April.

Barker, D. (1991) 'The foetal and infant origins of inequalities in health in Britain'. *Journal of Public Health Medicine*, 13: 64–8.

Bartley, M. (1994) 'Unemployment and ill health: understanding the relationship'. *Journal of Epidemiology and Community Health*, 48: 333–7.

Bartley, M., Blane, D. and Davey-Smith, G. (eds) (1998) *The Sociology of Health Inequalities*. Oxford: Blackwell.

Bauman, Z. (1998) *Globalization: The Human Consequences*. Cambridge: Polity Press.

—— (1998a) *Work, Consumerism and the New Poor*. Buckingham: Open University Press.

—— (1999) *In Search of Politics*. Cambridge: Polity Press.

Becker, H. (1998) *Tricks of the Trade*. Chicago, IL: University of Chicago Press.

Bhaskar, R. (1989) *The Possibility of Naturalism* (second edition). Hemel Hempstead: Harvester Wheatsheaf.

—— (1989a) *Reclaiming Reality: A Critical Introduction to Contemporary Philosophy*. London: Verso.

—— (1994) *Plato etc: The Problems of Philosophy and their Resolution*. London: Verso.

Blaxter, M. (1997) 'Whose fault is it? People's own conceptions of the reasons for health inequalities'. *Social Science and Medicine*, 44: 747–56.

Carchedi, G. (1977) *On the Economic Identification of Social Classes*. London: Routledge & Kegan Paul.

Chase-Dunn, C. (1989) *Global Formation: Structures of the World Economy*. Oxford: Blackwell.

Clement, W. and Myles, J. (1997) *Relations of Ruling: Class and Gender in Postindustrial Societies*. Montreal: McGill–Queen's University Press.

Cohen, J. and Arato, A. (1992) *Civil Society and Political Theory*. Cambridge, MA: MIT Press.

Collier, A. (1994) *Critical Realism: An Introduction to Roy Bhaskar's Philosophy*. London: Verso.

Crompton, R. (1998) *Class and Stratification* (second edition). Cambridge: Polity Press.

Dean, H. and Melrose, M. (1999) *Poverty, Riches and Social Citizenship*. London: Macmillan Press Ltd.

Denzin, N. (1989) *The Research Act* (third edition). Englewood Cliffs, NJ: Prentice-Hall.

Dhalgren, G. and Whitehead, M. (1991) *Policies and Strategies to Promote Social Equity in Health*. Stockholm: Institute for Future Studies.

Domhoff, G. (1967) *Who Rules America?* Englewood Cliffs, NJ: Prentice-Hall.

Doyal, L. (1979) *The Political Economy of Health*. London: Pluto Press.

—— (1995) *What Makes Women Sick? Gender and the Political Economy of Health*. London: Macmillan Press Ltd.

Drever, F. and Whitehead, M. (eds) (Office for National Statistics) (1997) *Health Inequalities*. Decennial Supplement. Series DS No 15. London: The Stationery Office.

Eichengreen, B. (1996) *Globalizing Capital: A History of the International Monetary System*. Princeton, NJ: Princeton University Press.

Elias, N. (1991) *The Society of Individuals*. Oxford: Blackwell.

—— (1996) *The Germans: Power Struggles and the Development of Habitus in the Nineteenth and Twentieth Centuries*. Cambridge: Polity Press.

Fraser, N. (1992) 'Rethinking the public sphere: a contribution to the critique of actually existing capitalism'. In Calhoun, C. (ed.) *Habermas and the Public Sphere*. Cambridge, MA: MIT Press.

Giddens, A. (1974) *Positivism and Sociology*. London: Heinemann.

Glaser, B. (1992) *Emergence vs. Forcing: Basics of Grounded Theory and Analysis*. Mill Valley, CA: Sociology Press.

Glaser, B. and Strauss, A. (1967) *The Discovery of Grounded Theory: Strategies for Qualitative Research*. Chicago, IL: Aldine.

Habermas, J. (1976) *Legitimation Crisis*. London: Heinemann.

—— (1984) *The Theory of Communicative Action, Volume One: Reason and the Rationalization of Society*. Cambridge: Polity Press.

—— (1987) *The Theory of Communicative Action, Volume Two: Lifeworld and System: A Critique of Functionalist Reason*. Cambridge: Polity Press.

—— (1991) 'Reply'. In Honneth, A. and Jones, A. (eds) *Communicative Action: Essays on Jürgen Habermas' The Theory of Communicative Action*. Cambridge, MA: MIT Press.

—— (1992) 'Concluding comments'. In Calhoun, C. (ed.) *Habermas and the Public Sphere*. Cambridge, MA: MIT Press.

—— (1996) *Between Facts and Norms: Contributions to a Discourse Theory of Law and Democracy*. Cambridge: Polity Press.

Held, D., McGrew, A., Goldblatt, D. and Perraton, J. (1999) *Global Transformations: Politics, Economics and Culture*. Cambridge: Polity Press.

Higgs, P. and Scambler, G. (1998) 'Explaining health inequalities: how useful are concepts of social class?' In Scambler, G. and Higgs, P. (eds) *Modernity, Medicine and Health: Medical Sociology Towards 2000*. London: Routledge.

Johnson, T., Dandeker, C. and Ashworth, C. (1984) *The Structure of Social Theory*. London: Macmillan Press Ltd.

Krieger, N. (1994) 'Epidemiology and the web of causation: has anyone seen the spider?' *Social Science and Medicine*, 39: 887–903.

Landes, D. (1998) *The Wealth and Poverty of Nations*. London: Little, Brown & Co.

Lash, S. and Urry, J. (1987) *The End of Organized Capitalism*. Cambridge: Polity Press.

Levinson, R. (1998) 'Issues at the interface of medical sociology and public health'. In Scambler, G. and Higgs, P. (eds) *Modernity, Medicine and Health: Medical Sociology Towards 2000*. London: Routledge.

Love, N. (1995) 'What's left of Marx?' In White, S. (ed.) *The Cambridge Companion to Habermas*. Cambridge: Cambrdge University Press.

Luhmann, N. (1982) *The Differentiation of Society*. New York: Columbia University Press.

—— (1995) *Social Systems*. Stanford, CA: Stanford University Press.

MacIntyre, S. and Hunt, K. (1997) 'Socio-economic position, gender and health: how do they interact?' *Journal of Health Psychology*, 2: 315–34.

Marmot, M., Davey-Smith, G., Stansfeld, S., Patel, C., North, F., Head, J., White, L., Brunner, E. and Feeney, A. (1991) 'Health inequalities among British civil servants: the Whitehall II Study'. *Lancet*, 37: 1387–93.

Marmot, M., Rose, G., Shipley, M. and Hamilton, P. (1978) 'Employment grade and coronary heart disease in British civil servants'. *Journal of Epidemiology and Community Health*, 3: 244–9.

Marshall, G., Newby, H., Rose, D. and Volger, C. (1988) *Social Class in Modern Britain*. London: Hutchinson.

McCarthy, T. (1984) 'Introduction'. In Habermas, J. *The Theory of Communicative Action,Volume One: Reason and the Rationalization of Society*. Cambridge: Polity Press.

Mills, C. Wright (1959) *The Sociological Imagination*. New York: Oxford University Press.

Nazroo, J. (1998) 'Genetic, cultural or socio-economic vulnerability? Explaining ethnic inequalities in health'. In Bartley, M., Blane, D. and Davey-Smith, G. (eds) *The Sociology of Health Inequalities*. Oxford: Blackwell.

Offe, C. (1985) *Disorganized Capitalism: Contemporary Transformations of Work and Politics*. Cambridge: Polity Press.

Popay, J., Williams, G., Thomas, C. and Gatrell, A. (1998) 'Theorizing inequalities in health: the place of lay knowledge'. In Bartley, M., Blane, D. and Davey-Smith, G. (eds) *The Sociology of Health Inequalities*. Oxford: Blackwell.

Popper, K. (1963) *Conjectures and Refutations*. London: Routledge & Kegan Paul.

—— (1972) *Objective Knowledge*. Oxford: Clarendon Press.

Rockmore, T. (1989) *Habermas on Historical Materialism*. Bloomington: Indiana University Press.

Scambler, G. (1998) 'Theorizing modernity: Luhmann, Habermas, Elias and new perspectives on health and healing'. *Critical Public Health*, 8: 237–44.

Scambler, G. and Higgs, P. (1999) 'Stratification, class and health: class relations and health inequalities in high modernity'. *Sociology*, 33: 275–96.

Scott, J. (1986) *Capitalists, Property and Financial Power*. Hassocks: Wheatsheaf.

—— (1991) *Who Rules Britain?* Cambridge: Polity Press.

—— (1996) *Stratification and Power: Structures of Class, Status and Command*. Cambridge: Polity Press.

—— (1997) *Corporate Business and Capitalist Classes*. Oxford: Oxford University Press.

Sitton, J. (1996) *Recent Marxian Theory: Class Formation and Social Conflict in Contemporary Capitalism*. New York: State University of New York Press.

—— (1998) 'Disembodied capitalism: Habermas' conception of the economy'. *Sociological Forum*, 13: 61–83.

Sklair, L. (1995) *Sociology of the Global System* (second edition). Baltimore, MD: Johns Hopkins University Press.

—— (1998) 'The transnational class'. In Carrier, J. and Miller, D. (eds) *Virtualism: A New Political Economy*. Oxford: Berg.

Smith, R. (1987) *Unemployment and Health: A Disaster and a Challenge*. Oxford: Oxford University Press.

Soros, G. (1998) *The Crisis of Global Capitalism: Open Society Endangered*. London: Little, Brown & Co.

Stationery Office (1998) *Report of the Independent Inquiry into Inequalities in Health* (Acheson Report). London: Stationery Office.

Strauss, A. and Corbin, J. (1990) *Basics of Qualitative Research: Grounded Theory Procedures and Techniques*. Newbury Park, CA: Sage.

Syme, S. (1996) 'To prevent disease: the need for a new approach'. In Blane, D., Brunner, E. and Wilkinson, R. (eds) *Health and Social Organization*. London: Routledge.

Therborn, G. (1978) *What does the Ruling Class do when it Rules?* London: New Left Books.

Useem, M. (1984) *The Inner Circle: Large Corporations and the Rise of Business Political Activity in the US and UK*. New York: Oxford University Press.

van Krieken, R. (1998) *Norbert Elias*. London: Routledge.

Wallerstein, E. (1998) *Utopistics: Or, Historical Choices of the Twenty-First Century*. New York: The New Press.

Warburton, P. (1999) *Debt and Delusion: Central Bank Follies that Threaten Economic Disaster*. London: Allen Lane.

Whitehead, M. (1995) 'Tackling inequalities: a review of policy initiatives'. In Benzeval, M., Judge, K. and Whitehead, M. (eds) *Tackling Inequalities in Health*. London: The King's Fund.

Willer, D. and Willer, J. (1973) *Systematic Empiricism: A Critique of a Pseudo-Science*. Englewood Cliffs, NJ: Prentice-Hall.

Williams, D., Lavizzo-Mourey, R. and Warren, R. (1994) 'The concept of race and health status in America'. *Public Health Reports*, 109: 26–41.

Chapter 6

New social movements in the health domain

David Kelleher

Introduction

'New social movements' have been a topic of interest both politically and sociologically since the 1960s. The term has been applied to a wide range of groups including those concerned with environmental issues, the women's movement in various forms, political groups which have been described as terrorists because of the methods they use to publicize their aims, and to groups like self-help groups whose aims are often thought of as personal. Although there is a wide variation in the aims, values and methods of those groups which are, from time to time, described as new social movements, sociologists have found it useful to use this generic label before attempting to look at differences between the groups. They have been described in a number of ways.

Offe (1985) sees the new social movements as being new in that they are not addressing the same problems as the 'old social movements' which were concerned essentially with class struggle. The liberal democratic states had learned to accept the old movements in the form of trade unions and collective bargaining and the various forms of the welfare state to achieve social control and manage conflicts in the wider political sphere.

> By the end of the fifties, the issues and proponents of socialism, neutralism, national unity, citizenship and economic democracy were reduced to virtual insignificance.
>
> (Offe, 1985: 824)

Although he describes the new social movements as being mainly concerned with 'way of life' issues he still sees them as political but to do with 'non-institutional politics'. In his discussion he considers the 'four most important ones' and identifies the issues which concern them, their values, modes of action and actors. Later, in discussing important values, he emphasizes these as being 'autonomy and identity (with their organizational correlates such as decentralization, self-government, and self-help) and opposition to manipulation, control, dependence, bureaucratization, regulation etc' (Offe, 1985: 829). Offe also supports the point made by Habermas (1987) that in contemporary capitalist society people experience deprivation in the consumer role as much as in their work role.

Not only is there wide agreement that the aims, values, methods and actors of new social movements vary enormously, but as Ray, drawing on Melucci (1989: 208–9), points out their visibility varies over time: 'social movements are "the nomads of the present", "submerged networks and laboratories of experience" where new answers are invented and tested' (Ray, 1993: 60).

Ray again refers to Melucci to suggest that new social movements are 'loosely bound, sympathetic friendship networks, involving consciousness raising, and opportunities to reconstruct life-histories ... where the formation of identities is more central than specific aims or objectives' (Ray, 1993: 61).

Some of the descriptive phrases which may be seen as being particularly relevant to self-help groups, although not directly in the way that Offe perhaps means, are those which suggest that these groups are seen as part of a new social movement, are often concerned with autonomy and identity, and opposition to control and dependence. The description of them as being 'sympathetic friendship networks, involving consciousness raising' providing the opportunities for the re-formation of identities is more directly applicable as will be suggested later.

Why have they developed?

Self-help groups in the domain of medicine have been growing in popularity in England and are even more numerous in continental Europe and the USA (Kelleher, 1994). What, then, has brought into focus since the 1960s so many forms of new social movement, and in particular the self-help groups which will be discussed in more detail later in this chapter?

Eyerman and Jamison (1991) consider a number of approaches which sociologists have used to try to understand the rise of the new social movements of the twentieth century and note how particularly unsatisfactory the explanations offered for the student movement of the 1960s have been. They takes the view that in the main European sociologists have suggested that the growth of new social movements reflects not only strains in the historical development of western society but also some possible ways in which the system might benefit from their development. Habermas is seen as an example of how new social movements can be understood in this way, as coming into being as a result not so much of the development of different forms of knowledge, which he discusses in *Knowledge and Human Interests* (1972), but as a result of the separation of technical, expert knowledge from lifeworld knowledge and practices. New social movements such as the ecological groups may then come into being as a means of attempting to build links between the different human interests and forms of knowledge. White quotes from an article by Habermas to show new social movements in this positive way:

> Rather the question is how to defend or reinstate endangered ways of life, or how to put reformed ways of life into practice. In short the new conflicts are not sparked by problems of distribution, but concern the grammar of forms of life.
>
> (White, 1989: 123)

White goes on to argue that in his view Habermas provides the most satisfactory and well-developed argument to account for the rise of new social movements, and also the 'best framework ... for constructing explanations of the behavior of new social movements' (White, 1989: 124) and the best means of understanding the work that they do. The way in which groups operate will be examined later in this chapter by looking at the example of self-help groups, but in terms of why they have arisen White makes the point that 'from Habermas' perspective, new social movements are reacting against the increasing colonization of the life-world and cultural impoverishment' (White, 1989: 124).

It is important though to explain briefly what is meant by the terms 'colonization' and 'cultural impoverishment'. For Habermas the term colonization means here not that it is the rationalization of the lifeworld as such which is seen as pathological, but the fact that it is instrumental rationality that has seeped into the lifeworld in ways which may be presented as beneficial, such as in the bureaucratization or 'juridification' of the welfare state, but which have in the process turned active citizens into 'clients'. As clients, they receive their due benefits but do not join with their fellow citizens in playing a part in the discussion of public issues surrounding the range of new treatments for conditions such as infertility and, in the process, become integrated into society. The only judgements being made in the operation of the various branches of the welfare state in a colonized world become technical ones about efficiency, to the exclusion of lifeworld moral and political issues. Similarly, the term 'cultural impoverishment' refers not to a decline in 'the arts' but to a reduction in the public sphere, in the capability of the lifeworld to perform the socially integrative functions of passing on and creating values; and to a reduction of 'communicative action' and the processes of joint identity construction in which it will be suggested later new social movements come to play a part.

Although a number of theorists (Eyerman and Jamison, 1991; Ray, 1993) offer explanations of why new social movements have come into being, it is, as will be argued later, Habermas who seems most convincing in offering an approach which suggests not only why they come into being but also how they can be seen as a positive response to the pressures of colonization and cultural deprivation. An examination of the role of self-help groups in the domain of medicine offers an example of both what brings them into being and how they can be seen as a creative response, not just a defence, against the excessive 'healthism' (Glassner, 1989) in contemporary society which makes chronically ill people feel not only stigmatized but to blame for their condition. It also provides an alternative to seeing self-help groups as being, like the television shows which invite 'confessionals', a means of engaging in a post-modern drive for intimacy.

New social movements in the domain of medicine cannot be said to be addressing political issues in a direct sense. It will be argued, however, that they are a political phenomenon in terms of the contribution they make to communicative action and, in so doing, promoting not just important integrative processes in resisting the colonization of the lifeworld by experts but in sustaining debates in a part of the public sphere.

Self-help groups as a new social movement

An area in which self-help groups have made a considerable contribution has been mental health. User groups, as they have been called in this area of the health domain, have been described by Pilgrim and Rogers (1993; Rogers and Pilgrim, 1991) as being part of a new social movement. They also note that such groups are more common in Europe and the USA than in England. Other accounts of self-help groups range from those to do with the users of tranquillizer drugs (Tattersall and Hallstrom, 1992; Gabe, 1994), to one which describes how a self-help group enabled people with epilepsy to feel more in control of their condition (Arntson and Droge, 1987), to those for people with psoriasis (Jobling, 1988). The World Health Organization (WHO) has seen them as important enough to publish summaries of the general features of self-help groups (see Kaplun, 1992). Some groups such as the Trigeminal Neuralgia Association in the USA are linked into a network and operate as a pressure group on medical authorities as well as offering support at a local level. Frank (1989: 160) points out the interesting example of AIDS groups which he says make claims (validity claims) which 'are not specific to themselves, but can be generalised to all ill persons'. Most of these articles describe what the groups do for the individuals who attend them, giving social support for example, and American studies sometimes refer to how they may also help communities (Reissman, 1997; Gartner and Reissman, 1998). A more extended description of what happens in self-help groups will be given later.

There are also attempts to explain how they have come into being in the medical domain. Some make an attempt to explain the emergence of the groups by referring to the shortcomings, in terms of caring, in the medical domain and Rogers and Pilgrim (1991) refer to the work of Offe (1984) in seeing new social movements in general as part of a political process which marginalized sections of a welfare economy employ to represent their interests. In their 1993 book, they also refer to Habermas to make the debatable point that the user groups are a 'new' social movement because they 'seek to establish new agendas and conquer new territory' rather than to 'defend existing social and property rights from erosion by the state' (Pilgrim and Rogers, 1993: 173). Scambler (1987) makes a brief reference to Habermas in suggesting that several women's groupings such as the Maternity Alliance are examples of user groups which, while remaining 'at the level of particularistic demands', can be seen as part of the women's movement, a new social movement of an 'offensive progressive' kind. A slightly more developed attempt to use the ideas of Habermas to understand self-help groups as being part of a new social movement was made by Kelleher (1994), and the rest of this chapter will develop that preliminary outline.

An outline of the theory of Habermas in relation to self-help groups

A starting point for Habermas in his general theory is Weber's concept of rationality and the beginnings of the idea that separate areas of world cultural value spheres had different forms of rationality. Drawing on Weber, Habermas identifies three such separate domains – science and technology; morality and law; art and literature – all three of which have their own forms of rationality or argumentation, but in his detailed critique of Weber's theory of rationality, Habermas wants to extend the concept of rationality to include the practices of everyday life:

> To the degree that the institutionalized production of knowledge that is specialized according to cognitive, normative, and aesthetic validity claims penetrates to the level of everyday communication and replaces traditional knowledge in its interaction-guiding functions, there is a rationalization of everyday practice ... a rationalization of the lifeworld that Weber neglected ...
>
> (Habermas, 1991: 340)

What is also important is that for Habermas rationalization does not always refer to the purposive instrumental form of rationality, although this is a form of rationalization which does invade and distort activities of the lifeworld by various processes. In Habermas' view of lifeworld rationalization, the validity of traditional knowledge, moral expectations and practices of sociation may be challenged in the processes of communicative action. There is a freeing of values from institutions and of moral expectations from the mores of culture, space for personalities to develop in modern society and therefore greater need to recognize the ways in which cultural changes become legitimated by processes of argumentation in the lifeworld. Concerning the processes of argumentation, which constitute rationality and which take place in the lifeworld, Habermas makes several critical theoretical assumptions. Central to the concept of communicative action is the theory of universal pragmatics, which draws on the ideas of Chomsky, Austin and Searle, and a consideration of the nature of speech acts. What is important here is that embedded in the notion of universal pragmatics is the assumption that competent speakers master not just 'rules for the generation of sentences in any language' but competence in mastering 'pragmatic rules that form the infrastructure of speech situations in general' (McCarthy, 1984: 279), that is, the ability to produce speech appropriate to the context. As White, commenting on Habermas, states:

> His claim is that the speech acts of communicatively competent actors conform to a set of rules, some of which establish the criteria of communicative rationality.
>
> (White, 1989: 28)

And Habermas makes the further claim that

> By attending to the modes of language use, we can clarify what it means to a speaker, in performing one of the standard speech acts, to take up a pragmatic relation
> – to something in the objective world ...
> – to something in the social world ...
> – to something in the subjective world (as the totality of experience to which a speaker has privileged access to and which he can express before a public).
>
> (Habermas, 1987: 120)

Such a view of language use is implicit in Habermas' understanding of the normal utterances of people engaged in activities of the lifeworld. But it is necessary also to explain what is meant by 'normal'. The important thing about his claim concerning the rationality of the lifeworld is that in the normal utterances of communicative action people are intersubjectively able to reach agreement or define the basis of their disagreement if the hearer accepts the truth of the statement being made, accepts it as being valid to express such a statement in the normative framework of the situation, and accepts that the speaker is speaking sincerely. The ability to assess the validity of statements is learned as part of the ability, as is the ability to detect insincerity or irony where, says Habermas, we recognize that there is an intention to go against the normal. White is doubtful about this ability to see through the ideological use of language and raises a number of criticisms of Habermas' concept of 'normal'.

> His privileging of serious, straightforward, unambiguous usage can be seen as diverting our attention away from precisely those aspects of language which have the capability of sensitizing us to the oppressiveness of whatever categorial distinctions are dominating our thought and social interaction in any given historical period.
>
> (White, 1989: 31)

While this is an important point, it is not a damning criticism of relevance to our consideration of self-help groups.

One other point needs to be made about Habermas' view of language before considering communicative action and the lifeworld in slightly more detail and prior to going on to relate these concepts to self-help groups in the domain of medicine. Habermas sees narration as a special form of statement-making which helps people not only communicate with others but also to understand themselves:

> Narrative practice not only serves trivial needs for mutual understanding ... it also has a function in the self-understanding of persons ... they can develop personal identities only if they recognise that the sequences of their own actions form narratively presentable life histories; they can develop social identities only if they recognize that they maintain their membership in social groups by way of participating in interactions ...
>
> (Habermas, 1987: 136)

It will be argued below that this function of language use which Habermas describes has relevance for analysing the activities of self-help groups.

Communicative action is oriented to actors reaching understanding. As Habermas outlines it:

communicative action serves to transmit and renew cultural knowledge; under the aspect of coordinating action, it serves social integration and the establishment of solidarity; finally, under the aspect of socialization, communicative action serves the formation of personal identities.

(Habermas, 1987: 137)

The communicative model is based on Habermas' concepts of speech acts and the already mentioned ability of speakers/listeners to rationally and intersubjectively define the situation, to speak truly and to reach agreement or to understand the basis of their disagreement. There is an important condition which is hypothesized in this model, which is that for such an exchange of argumentation to occur there must be 'an ideal speech situation'. This means that the actors must have no constraints, either conscious or unconscious, and no sense of being dominated in the processes of reaching agreement; all participants must have an equal opportunity to contribute. As McCarthy notes,

the space–time limitations, the psychological and other limitations of actual discourse seem to preclude a perfect realization of these conditions. Nonetheless this does not of itself render the ideal illegitimate, an ideal that can be more or less adequately approximated in reality, that can serve as a guide for the institutionalization of discourse and as a critical standard against ...

(McCarthy, 1984: 309)

Although the ideal speech situation is an ideal which is never realized in real situations it can be used to discuss the features of actual situations to see whether they approximate to or diverge from the ideal.

The lifeworld is the last concept to look at before going on to consider how self-help groups might be seen as an example of a new social movement. Habermas uses both Parsons and Marx in his structural analysis of society. He sees the rationalization of society which Weber had described as taking place in a system with a number of subsystems. He is critical of social theory which suggests that society can be understood as a complex, self-regulating system which is maintained and developed by rational processes. He has developed his own critical theory of historical evolution by attempting to overcome what he sees as the limitations of systems theory, which has a limited notion of social action, and incorporating the contributions of various hermeneutic approaches (see ch. 3 in McCarthy, 1984). In taking up the question of social action Habermas draws firstly on Durkheim and Mead. He begins by noting the 'unclarified relation between action theory and systems theory' (Habermas, 1987: 113) and goes on to say,

> It is not Durkheim's answer but the way he poses the question that is instructive. It directs our attention to empirical connections between stages of system differentiation and forms of social integration ... No matter whether one starts with Mead from basic concepts of social interaction or with Durkheim from basic concepts of collective representation, in either case society is conceived from the perspective of acting subjects as the lifeworld of a social group.
>
> (Habermas, 1987: 117)

In constructing his own critical theory of historical evolution Habermas has drawn on a wide range of other theories and he is aware of the limitations of hermeneutic theories, as well as the system ones, but he wants to include an action theory which is based on the lifeworld.

I would like therefore to propose :

> (1) that we conceive of societies simultaneously as systems and lifeworlds.
>
> (Habermas, 1987: 118)

In explicating the concept of lifeworld he points out the links with formal pragmatics, speech acts and communicative action. Unusually for Habermas, in illustrating the concept of the lifeworld he works through an example showing what the group of building workers, including the new recruit, would already need to share as part of their lifeworld, in an imagined situation of the builders asking the new recruit to go for the mid-morning refreshment (Habermas, 1987: 121). They would already share as part of their common lifeworld assumptions a definition of the situation, the appropriateness of the task or theme (fetching the beer) and the normative acceptability of the new recruit being asked by the older workers to perform this task. All would recognize that the request was a sincere one (unlike the kind of request which is intended to make a fool of the recruit by sending him to get some striped paint).

Language and culture and assumptions of what is appropriate in particular contexts are shown to be part of the background of the lifeworld in which people communicatively interact, and these provide speakers and listeners with common background convictions which they use in reaching understandings but which also allow them to negotiate new understandings in changing situations.

> The lifeworld is, so to speak, the transcendental site where speaker and hearer meet, where they can reciprocally raise claims that their utterances fit the world (objective, social, or subjective), and where they can criticize and confirm those validity claims, settle their disagreements, and arrive at agreements.
>
> (Habermas, 1987: 126)

In the process of communicative interaction in the lifeworld people are not simply reaching agreement however; they are also engaging in the integrative process of renewing their activity as members of groups and affirming their own identities.

In the theory of Habermas the lifeworld is an important part of society; it is also important that system and lifeworld remain integrated, for the mechanisms of the system, such as the free market economy and the legal system, need to be anchored in the values of the lifeworld. As the system becomes more differentiated and the lifeworld more rationalized, there is a risk of 'uncoupling'. This may happen through developments within the total system such as bureaucratization, and the development of powerful economic blocs and of expert systems. All of these may use instrumental-purposive rationality, thus side-stepping, by use of the steering *mechanisms* of power and money, the linguistified consensus-reaching ways of the lifeworld and the moral-practical elements which are an essential part of lifeworld considerations.

The political link between system and lifeworld is the public sphere, which is the territory in which new social movements operate.

Medicine, as Scambler discusses in his essay 'Habermas and the power of medical expertise' (Scambler, 1987), has become an enormously powerful expert system which manages many conditions and situations in ways which take them out of the public sphere to a place where the appropriateness of medical definitions can be challenged. Scambler's example is built around the experience of childbirth, but other conditions such as the menopause, infertility and hyperactivity have all been seen as examples of 'medicalization', or the removal of issues from discussion in the public sphere, where questions of a moral-practical nature might be asked. Using Habermas' theory, these could all be understood as cases in which the limited purposive-instrumental rationality which dominates expert systems 'colonizes the lifeworld'. The values and concerns and the communicative interactive style of reaching understanding of the lifeworld are set aside and treatments and what counts as success are decided by expert practitioners.

Scambler (1987), in introducing his argument that medical knowledge, based as it is in science and technology, has come to overpower the lay knowledge of childbirth possessed by women, suggests that this can be seen as an example of the colonization of the lifeworld. The purposive-rational action has, in the illustrative exchanges between doctor and expectant mother, been used to over-rule her lifeworld concerns. He also draws attention to the way the concept of 'compliance' is used in studies of doctor–patient interaction; only patients are seen as non-compliant. They are described by doctors as non-compliant if they do not follow the treatment and behaviour recommended by the doctor, but, as Mishler (1984) and others have argued, the non-compliance of patients may be the result of one-sided consultations in which the 'voice of the lifeworld' has been ignored. In a study of diabetic patients and 'non-compliance', Kelleher (1988) suggests that doctors tend to label as 'difficult' people who want to incorporate their own experiential knowledge of diabetes into the management of their condition. Scambler (1987: 179) sees such studies as reflecting 'the current imbalance between system rationalization and the rationalization of the lifeworld ... '.

Two related points can be made by his references to studies of medical consultations: first, many studies make the point that medical consultations are far from being 'ideal speech situations' in which agreement is reached about how to manage a chronic condition by a reciprocal exchange of statements and questioning in communicative interaction; secondly, although some people are willing to accept the advice of the 'expert', a number of others feel dissatisfied and in various ways want to resist medical control. It is suggested that this resistance can be understood as an example of the way in which some kinds of self-help groups come into being: there may be a setting in which the knowledge of experts becomes more open to the critical capacities of lay people, a developing part of the public sphere.

If we look at what self-help groups are and what they do we can see to what extent they can be understood in this way. Most writers agree that there is considerable variation between groups. Vincent (1992) suggests that there is a continuum.

> At one pole are self-help groups which conform to the 'ideal type' or model in which all are therapists, offering reciprocal care and support; along the continuum come groups in which only some members take the therapeutic role and/or responsibility for the tasks of the group; then come groups which offer services in a traditional way, that is given by the few to those defined as deserving (in this case only to their members); finally, at the opposite pole are groups which may retain a core of self-help but whose main activity is providing services in the mould of a traditional voluntary organization.
>
> (Vincent, 1992: 144)

She goes on to say that

> they involve members as responsible persons ... and the individualization of disease and the power of professionals is called into question.
>
> (Vincent, 1992: 145)

Williams (1989) describes the historical development of the idea of self-help before going on to examine the nature of one group. He sees the National Ankylosing Spondylitis Society as torn by tensions between those who think that it should be

> a patients' society for teaching the medical and caring professions what their [patients'] problems really are ... those who see it as a friendly support group, and those who want it to be 'a prestigious charitable society'.
>
> (Williams, 1989: 146)

Kelleher (1994) surveys a range of descriptions and definitions including the oft-used definiton of Katz and Bender (1976), which divides self-help groups into those in which the main activity is members sharing their problems and supporting one another, which Katz and Bender call 'inner-focussed' groups, and those whose main activity is acting as a pressure group to improve facilities for people with that particular condition, which they call 'outer-focussed'. He reports that Robinson and Henry (1977: 141) conclude that self-help groups are not a political phenomenom but 'people who are coming together to share and solve their common problems, rather than put up with the frustrations and humiliations of professional services'.

When we look at what people say self-help groups enable people to do, we find ideas range from what some doctors think – allow 'people to let off steam' (Kelleher, 1990) – to Trojan's 1989 German study, in which he says they allow people to gain new knowledge and give them the confidence to express themselves, to those which emphasize the fact that they give people the opportunity to incorporate their illness condition into their identity. Both Williams (1989) and Arntson and Droge (1987) make this point. Williams refers to the usefulness of the process of 'narrative reconstruction' and Arntson and Droge (1987: 153) say: 'self-help group members provide each other with the opportunities, stories and sets of behaviors in order to increase their perceived control over their physical and social conditions'.

Stewart, in a review article, although she is particularly concerned with describing the 'interface' between professionals and groups, also summarizes a number of the functions which self-help groups perform. She suggests that as well as providing mutual support they empower members by increasing their confidence and competence. They also bring into question the professionals' beliefs: 'Clearly, self-help groups and other social movements bring the individualistic bias of professionals into question' (Stewart, 1990: 1155). Later she recommends that students in the healthcare field need to learn that expert solutions should not always take precedence over experiential solutions. Kelleher (1994) also concludes that one of the important functions of self-help groups is that they help members to feel more confident about their experiential knowledge and to 'challenge and interrogate' medical knowledge. One example he gives of this from an observational study of eight groups for people with diabetes is that when animal-based insulin was being replaced by genetically engineered 'human' insulin a number of people reported difficulties such as getting no warning when they were 'going hypo'. When they had individually reported this in medical consultations, their complaints tended to be dismissed in terms of them just 'not liking something new'; when their experiences were confirmed by others in self-help groups they gained the confidence to complain further through the British Diabetic Association (BDA) who then got an 'expert' inquiry set up and, subsequently, guidelines on the matter were issued to consultants. This issue was revived in the *Guardian* in March 1999 (see Brown, 1999) when it was suggested that a report on people's experiences of changing over to the new form of insulin had been withheld from publication. A letter from the BDA's research director in the newspaper the following day explained that it had not been published because it was simply a compilation of the views of 380 diabetic people and it was 'not scientific' – an interesting comment on the importance attached to the views of patients. A comparison between the 'branches' of the national association (BDA), which has evolved since being set up by people with diabetes in the 1920s, and the self-help groups set up in the late 1980s is itself interesting. It shows how user groups may become incorporated into the professional domain, for although the BDA does campaign on behalf of diabetic people and branches do provide a place for friendships to be made, much of the time is taken up by professionals giving advice and by fundraising activities. The important committees of the BDA are also led by professionals. The moving spirits behind the setting up of the self-help groups wanted to free themselves from fundraising activities and professional domination to provide 'inner-focussed' support for members.

Another part of the health domain where there have been radical groups of a political kind set up has been in the area of mental illness. Rogers and Pilgrim (1991) state that in this area at least it could be argued that a 'patients' view' which is different from, and in some ways in opposition to, the views of professionals has developed. They see the mental health user groups that they are interested in as part of a 'new social movement' and draw on definitions by Toch and Habermas to support this claim. Their interest is in those groups which engage in political campaigning rather than in those user-led groups which offer support in a self-help way, 'even though they might regard themselves justifiably as part of the movement' (Rogers and Pilgrim, 1991: 132).

An interesting example of the political campaigning type of group which they give is the campaign waged by user groups in 1988 against the proposed amendment to the 1983 Mental Health Act. This amendment to community treatment orders would have allowed doctors to treat patients in the community on a compulsory basis. The objection lay in the use of physical treatments, which they abhorred, in the community; it was an example of collectively resisting the extension of professional control into the everyday lives of users.

Still in the mental health domain but looking at a unique users' group which is concerned with the personal lives of members is a study by Shoenberg (1994). This is a study of six people in a 'drop in centre' run by users for users and from which professionals were excluded except on one day a week. Besides providing facilities such as a washing machine and rooms for relaxation and watching television, a range of activities were run by users; these included a 'hearing voices' group, an art group, an insomnia group and a 'survivors poetry performance' group. Although this study is primarily concerned with illustrating the views of individual users, the existence of such a centre under the control of users is an indication of their desire to share experiences and reach understandings outside of the control of professionals.

Linking concepts and practice

We can now see how the activities described above can be understood using the concepts and theory of Habermas. In the 'inner-focussed' groups one of the main activities of members is to better understand their condition in ways that make sense of their experience of it. They are not usually dismissing what they have learned about it from doctors and other healthcare professionals but they often feel that what they have experienced is dismissed by doctors. When they meet with others with the same condition they make the assumptions Habermas suggests would exist in an ideal speech situation, that is, that the others, like themselves, are sincere in what they say and are describing it truthfully in a way that is normatively appropriate for the context. That is not to suggest that all the conditions of ideal speech exist; it may be that although all members share the condition and are ostensibly equal, some members are coercive in that they speak in a way which is authoritative, and therefore, that other members feel they cannot challenge their accounts and hesitate to relate their different experience, thus negating one of the important aspects of the ideal speech situation. It is possible too that members may be inhibited by the setting of the meeting. In the observational study of diabetic self-help groups (Kelleher, 1991), those groups which met either in someone's home or on NHS property seemed less free-wheeling than those which met in a room in a public house or community centre. It may be useful therefore to use the concept of the ideal speech situation as a measure against which actual situations can be compared.

Reference has already been made to the value Habermas sees in the special kind of (constative) statement-making speech which is part of constructing a narrative. Although, as Mathieson and Stam (1995) warn in their article about cancer narratives, we should not take all stories constructed by individuals about themselves as being 'a narrative' and, as Habermas (1987: 137) himself points out, narrative is a lifeworld concept rather than a theoretical one, the latter does see narration as helping to achieve the lifeworld concern with integration: 'Collectivities maintain their identities only to the extent that the ideas members have of their lifeworld overlap sufficiently and condense into unproblematic background convictions' (Habermas, 1987: 136).

In the diabetic self-help group study already referred to (Kelleher, 1991), the training of the group leaders encouraged what was called 'personal' talk and in the groups observed they were always pleased when someone began on a life-history. An example of this was when a man in his early 40s who worked as a landscape gardener began to talk about how having recently become diabetic, he was experiencing difficulties in his marriage. He was obviously angry and wanted help in understanding what was happening to him and his life. He was listened to sympathetically and his talk prompted others to talk in a similar way about their own lives. In this way it could be said that not only were they coming to understand themselves but they were helping to construct a joint narrative about experiencing diabetes and gaining a feeling of being less like isolated sufferers and more of a feeling of solidarity with others. Their lifeworld assumptions of what it is to be a person, which had been shattered by learning that they had a chronic illness, were being reconstructed by sharing in the experiences of others.

Arntson and Droge (1987), in analysing their observations in self-help groups for people with epilepsy, have some interesting comments on the use of narration. It is apparent that to describe it as simply 'social support' is inadequate. They note the differences between what they call the 'dialectical' and hierarchical character of doctor–patient consultations and the often didactic nature of conversations with other family members, and contrast this with the freedom to 'suspend literal truth claims in order to draw a higher order truth about life' that narrators exerienced in the self-help group. Whether the characteristic of self-help groups' talk could be taken to represent the kind of questioning that Habermas would see as being part of the process of communicative interaction is not clear as they are not using a Habermasian framework to understand their data. From what is said about the narrations being made in a non-hierarchical context and helping the narrators to gain a sense of control over their epilepsy, however, it could be said that in so far as they are jointly re-constructing their identities as people with epilepy and as members of the group they are building on what have become the unexplicated lifeworld assumptions of people with epilepsy.

It seems that in these groups and in many non-professionally directed groups at least some of the features of communicative interaction are present. Members are engaged in talk with others which is helping them to re-construct their identities in ways in which, for some at least, their conditions are accepted. The groups are socially integrating in that they normalize for members the ways that most manage their condition. Until they hear that others manage the condition in a similar way, they have often felt, individually, like failures needing to apologize to the doctor for their non-compliance ('I've been a bit naughty, doctor') instead of having the confidence to talk about how the other priorities in their lives could be integrated with medical ones. The talk in the self-help groups is rational in the way that Habermas sees lifeworld talk as being the construction of meaning, and different from the means–ends, instrumentally rational kind of interaction that is often the pattern in consultations with professionals. The medical management of a condition such as diabetes, for example, is only partly about managing the present, avoiding hypoglycaemia or hyperglycaemia; it is concerned also with managing it to try to avoid the long-term complications of neuropathy, nephropathy and retinopathy.

In the groups the lifeworld assumptions which are part of people's everyday commonsense are used in linking their actual experiences of eating, working, having sexual relations, to their condition, whereas, as Mishler (1984) has suggested, these everyday experiences are made to seem irrelevant in medicine's pursuit of its own concerns in consultations. In firstly encouraging the development of rationality in the lifeworld by creating a communicative interaction style of talk and in bringing the rational understanding of lifeworld concerns into relations with the technical rationality of the subsystem of medicine by the discussion and comparison of experiences, self-help groups could be said to be resisting the uncoupling of system and lifeworld. They are also a means by which the colonization of the lifeworld is resisted in that the limited medical accounts of what it is to have diabetes/epilepsy etc. can be widened as the experiential knowledge of people, such as the lack of warning of changes from animal-based insulin to genetically engineered or other effects, is confirmed or rejected and shown to be valid or invalid. Either way the expert knowledge of medicine, with its instrumental rationality, becomes understood in ways that relate it to lifeworld concerns. If the only understanding that people have of their condition is the medical one then this comes to dominate the way they live, or feel they should live, and their lives are constrained by what are experienced as rigid treatment routines, to the exclusion of social relationships and even work. All people with a chronic illness are torn by how they should live, as sick people or as normal people who are managing a condition. If they come to see themselves as sick people, the demands of treatment routines dominate their lives and the ordinary lifeworld assumptions are pushed aside. It could be said that system values are dominating (colonizing) the lifeworld and such lifeworld functions as socialization and integration are diminished.

Limitations of self-help groups in the domain of medicine

It cannot be claimed that the groups described here are emancipatory or political in the narrow sense although Rogers and Pilgrim (1991) appear to want to do this. But Habermas (1987: 393) himself draws a distinction between such new social movements as the women's movement and other groups which have a more defensive character. 'The resistance and withdrawal movements aim at stemming formally organized domains of action for the sake of communicatively structured domains, and not at conquering new territory.'

The self-help groups described here then are not political in the sense that those new social movements campaigning to save the environment are, nor are they political in wanting to work for political change of the kind sought by the old social movements associated with labour. The argument that they are 'part of the culture of new social movements' is based on seeing them as, first, defending certain defined parts of the lifeworld from colonization by an expert system which itself has become dominated by the instrumental rationality of the larger system of society; and secondly, in that they make provision for the powerful knowledge of medicine to be challenged, they could be said to be contributing to sustaining a public sphere in a similar way to the new social movement groups which are overtly politicizing issues. There is no doubt, as Holub (1991) points out, that the public sphere is an important part of Habermas' work, something that he sees as vital in a democratic society with pluralist values, and one of the settings in which it can continue to operate is in those self-help groups in which the assumptions of the lifeworld, the cultural expectations about life, and the voice of medicine can be put side by side in ways which allow the powerful, instrumental rationality of medical experts to be challenged.

There is another sense in which self-help groups could be said to be political, and that is in the contribution they make to remedying one of the weaknesses in an important part of welfare states, which are themselves important either in contributing to the success of social democratic societies or in masking their limitations and so preventing real change from taking place, depending on the point of view taken. The contribution they make here is in providing patients with an opportunity to talk about their feelings about having a particular condition, something healthcare professionals seem unable to do. As Arntson and Droge (1987) note,

> For the practitioner, the health encounter is highly scripted, time limited ... Many encounters were finished in under a minute... Many epilepsy patients at the clinic were upset that they did not get to discuss other aspects of having epilepsy with the doctor.
>
> (Arntson and Droge, 1987: 158)

Similarly, in Kelleher's work (1991) 55 per cent of BDA members (a different group from the self-help group members) agreed with the statement 'Doctors don't encourage people to talk about their feelings' and only 11 per cent agreed with the statement that 'If you have a good doctor you don't need a self-help group'.

The unwillingness of healthcare professionals to spend time may be partly a result of shortage of time, as they claim, but it is also an example of how communication is structured by hierarchies of power, lifeworld concerns are excluded and interaction distorted. As Frank (1989: 359) says, doctors and nurses do not speak in 'validity claims' but in 'orders'.

The claim of self-help groups to be part of a new social movement is therefore a limited one, but evidence of what is going on in self-help groups in the medical domain does show that the people in them are beginning to act in a participatory style. This enables them to resist the bland definitions of themselves as consumers or clients which individualize their responses instead of allowing them to communicatively debate and challenge the limited nature of medical understandings. Habermas (1987: 395) suggests that 'It is above all in the domains of social policy and health policy (e.g. in connection with psychiatric care) that models of reform point in this direction'.

It is clear from such asides, and from his recent essay on the differences in the discourses on human rights in western and Asiatic cultures, that Habermas (1999) does intend his theoretical concepts to be used to reveal differences and promote debate, and although the part played by self-help groups may be small it is indicative of the way resistances can be made.

There are other limitations. The numbers of people in self-help groups are small in England and although more people attend them in continental Europe and in some they are integrated into the structure of the healthcare system, there is a danger that they will lose their challenging edge and become another means which professionals see of educating patients about their condition. As Frank (1989) says in discussing how Habermas takes us further than Mead in understanding how salesmen talk,

> For Habermas, the salesman is not acting communicately but strategically. The salesman seeks to define the situation so that only what he himself wants is plausible ... strategic action seeks only to convince, communicative action proceeds in a willingness to be convinced.
>
> (Frank, 1989: 356)

The way that communication in self-help groups develops is critically important in relation to any claim that they are a way of sustaining a public sphere. Leaders of the groups need to be trained not only to know how to create the opportunities and ambience for narration as part of the process of identity reconstruction and development, but also how to move from chit-chat to challenge. It also requires them to have some understanding of the place of such groups in modern society. As Frank goes on to say: 'the distinctively modern breakdown of the communicative is not a sum of individual failings. Rather it represents a structural condition of society' (Frank, 1989: 356).

It is important to note then that not all groups which are called self-help groups can be said to be engaging in the communicative activities which would allow them to be included in the category of self-help as described here as being part of a 'new social movement'; only those which are operating mainly to provide members with the opportunity to construct personal and joint narratives, by allowing them to relate accounts and then questioning them, are performing the tasks of re-socializing people to see themselves as normal people with diabetes/epilepsy/schizophrenia, and only they can be seen as engaged in resisting the colonization of the lifeworld.

References

Arntson, P. and Droge, D. (1987) 'Social support in self-help groups'. In Albrecht, T., Adelman, M. and Associates *Communicating Social Support*. Newbury Park, CA: Sage.

Brown, P. (1999) 'Diabetics not told of insulin risk'. *Guardian*, 9 March, p. 6.

Eyerman, R. and Jamison, A. (1991) *Social Movements: A Cognitive Approach*. Cambridge: Polity Press.

Frank, A. (1989) 'Habermas' interactionism: the micro–macro link to politics'. *Symbolic Interactionism*, 12, 2: 253–60.

Gabe, J. (1994) 'Promoting benzodiazepine withdrawal'. *Addiction*, 89: 1497–1504.

Gartner, A. and Reissman, F. (1998) 'Self-help'. *Social Policy*, Spring: 83–6.

Glassner, B. (1989) 'Fitness and the postmodern self'. *Journal of Health and Social Behavior*, 30: 180–91.

Habermas, J. (1972) *Knowledge and Human Interests*. London: Heinemann.

—— (1987) *The Theory of Communicative Action, Volume Two: Lifeworld and System: A Critique of Functionalist Reason*. Cambridge: Polity Press.

—— (1984) *The Theory of Communicative Action, Volume One: Reason and the Rationalization of Society.* Cambridge: Polity Press.

—— (1999) 'Remarks on legitimation through human rights'. *Philosophy and Social Criticism*, 24, 2/3: 157–71.

Holub, R. (1991) *Jürgen Habermas: Critic in the Public Sphere.* London: Routledge.

Jobling, R. (1988) 'The *experience* of psoriasis under treatment'. In Anderson, R. and Bury, M. (eds) *Living With Chronic Illness.* London: Unwin Hyman.

Kaplun. A. (ed.) (1992) *Health Promotion and Chronic Illness.* Copenhagen: World Health Organization.

Katz, A. and Bender, E. (1976) *The Strength in Us.* New York: New Viewpoints.

Kelleher, D. (1988) 'Coming to terms with diabetes: coping strategies and non-compliance'. In Anderson, R. and Bury, M. (eds) *Living With Chronic Illness.* London: Unwin Hyman.

—— (1990) 'Do self-help-groups help?' *International Disability Studies*, 12: 66–9.

—— (1991) 'Patients learning from each other: self-help groups for people with diabetes'. *Journal of the Royal Society of Medicine*, 84: 595–7.

—— (1994) 'Self-help groups and their relationship to medicine'. In Gabe, J., Kelleher, D. and Williams, G. (eds) *Challenging Medicine.* London: Routledge.

Mathieson, C. and Stam, H. (1995) 'Renegotiating identity: cancer narratives'. *Sociology of Health and Illness*, 17, 3: 283–306.

McCarthy, T. (1984) *The Critical Theory of Jürgen Habermas.* Cambridge: Polity Press.

Melucci, A (1989) *Nomads of the present: Social movements and individual needs in contemporary society.* London; Hutchinson Radius.

Mishler, E. (1984) *The Discourse of Medicine: Dialectics of Medical Interviews.* Norwood, NJ: Ablex.

Offe, C. (1984) *Contradictions of the Welfare State.* London: Hutchinson.

—— (1985) 'New social movements: challenging the boundaries of institutional politics'. *Social Research*, 52: 817–68.

Pilgrim, D. and Rogers, A. (1993) *A Sociology of Mental Health and Illness.* Milton Keynes: Open University Press.

Ray, L. (1993) *Rethinking Critical Theory.* London: Sage.

Reissman, F. (1997) 'Ten self-help principles'. *Social Policy*, Spring: 6–11.

Robinson, D. and Henry, S. (1977) *Self-help and Health: Mutual Aid for Modern Problems.* London: Martin Robertson.

Rogers, A. and Pilgrim, D. (1991) 'Pulling down churches: accounting for the British mental health users' movement'. *Sociology of Health and Illness*, 13, 2: 129–48.

Scambler, G. (1987) 'Habermas and the power of medical expertise'. In Scambler, G. (ed.) *Sociological Theory and Medical Sociology*, London: Tavistock.

Shoenberg, H. (1994) *Interviewing Mental Health Users*. Unpublished MSc dissertation. London: London Guildhall University.

Stewart, M. (1990) 'Professional interface with mutual-aid self-help groups: a review'. *Social Science and Medicine*, 31, 10: 1143–58.

Tattersall, M. and Hallstrom, C. (1992) 'Self-help and benzodiazepine withdrawal'. *Journal of Affective Disorders*, 24: 193–8.

Trojan, A. (1989) 'Benefits of self-help groups: a survey of 232 members from 65 disease-related groups'. *Social Science and Medicine*, 29: 25–32.

Vincent, J. (1992) 'Self-help groups and healthcare in contemporary Britain'. In Saks, M. (ed.) *Alternative Medicine in Britain*. Oxford: Clarendon Press.

White, S. K. (1989)*The Recent Work of Jürgen Habermas: Reason, Justice and Modernity*. Cambridge: Cambridge University Press.

Williams, G. (1989) 'Hope for the humblest? The role of self-help in chronic illness: the case of ankylosing spondylitis'. *Sociology of Health and Illness*, 11, 2: 135–59.

Chapter 7

Finite resources and infinite demand

Public participation in health care rationing

Paul Higgs and Ian Rees Jones

Introduction

This chapter examines the emergence of health care rationing as an issue of public debate. In particular, it seeks to show how such a debate offers a false promise of democratic policy making that seems to accord with aspects of Habermas' ideal speech situation. We argue that attempts to gain public agreement and involvement regarding the principles underpinning decisions about resource allocation in health care do not meet the criteria for undistorted communication and therefore reflect underlying power relationships and indeed may replicate them. More importantly, we would argue, debates concerning criteria for rationing do not necessarily represent a positive way forward for empowering the general population but, rather, could represent a colonization of lifeworld values that have to date resisted such rationalization. We conclude that most attempts to create socially acceptable criteria for the rationing of health care services are doomed to replicate system-world priorities because of the way that they are set up. We further argue that in attempting to place health policy on a rational footing insufficient attention has been given to the processes and interests created by the operation of ideology in class societies.

We begin this chapter by tracing the various discourses on health care rationing in the public sphere. We go on to examine the contradictions that exist between professional and public views of rationing and how this has given rise to technical solutions to the 'problem' of rationing. We then subject the debate to an analysis based on a reading of Weberian and Habermasian concepts of rationality before introducing the importance of ideology for any attempt to democratize rationing through communicative practices of rationalization.

Rationing in the public sphere

Health care rationing is not a new phenomenon. As Ellen Annandale (1998) points out, present-day rationing dilemmas are uncannily presaged in George Bernard Shaw's play *The Doctor's Dilemma* published in 1911. Rationing therefore has been present in health care systems, whatever their form, for a very long time (Harrison and Moran, 2000). However, within the context of seemingly de-politicized and converging welfare systems, the technical question of meeting apparently infinite demands with limited budgets has become a *defining* issue. Rationing of health services as an issue filled the pages of the medical press throughout the 1990s, with leaders of the medical and managerial professions calling for an end to politicians' silence on this issue. Rationing was presented as the unavoidable nettle to grasp in any publicly funded health care system. Axiomatic was the view that there were not enough resources to meet the health care needs of all citizens and that some form of rationing was therefore inevitable (New, 1996). This position is now so widely accepted that it forms the orthodox position in health policy circles.

What accounts for this paradigm shift? After all the NHS was founded upon very different principles, tenets related to the notions of citizenship and the need for protection from the effects of markets. A conventional argument is that the founders of the NHS did not understand that they were seeking to do the impossible. The meeting of everybody's needs is impossible because as fast as old needs are met new ones come up to replace them – all the time demanding more and more resources. This dilemma, known as the 'Beveridge fallacy', forms the starting point for the rationing debate. The post-Second World War development of the British NHS was marked by difficulties over resourcing; however, these were put into second place by the need to create a rationalized organization for service delivery. The 1960s and 1970s were more notable for structural change than debates over the impossibility of meeting needs. Indeed, the change from planning to financing which accompanied the Callaghan government's introduction of cash limits was initially seen as an expedient rather than a revelation. The consolidation of neo-liberal thought into public policy was achieved by the post-1979 Conservative governments (Higgs, 1993). The explicit identification of public expenditure as a liability for economic growth saw the government embark on programmes of resource cutback, privatization and the marketization of public services. None of this meant that an explicit policy of rationing was about to be enacted. Far from it. During the 1980s and 1990s successive Conservative governments attempted to avoid such a conclusion by introducing clearer management and an element of competition into the financing and delivery of NHS services. All of this was done against a background of how to balance increasing health care costs with a commitment to lower the size of the tax burden. When the obvious contradictions of this aspiration became apparent and recurring 'NHS crises' happened, the blame was placed at the feet of systemic inefficiency, bad management or a lack of consumer orientation. Rationing as an explicit policy smacked of state control and the politicization of need, while the chosen mechanism of change – an internal or bounded market – offered an alternative. Because markets are deemed to be in the business of matching supply with demand and in the process creating an efficient use of resources the difficulties necessitating rationing would be overcome.

Obviously, as many commentators were aware, the introduction of an internal market in the 1990s did not solve the problem of resourcing the NHS; rather, it moved the responsibility for decision making away from the government. It would still be necessary for managers to prioritize between services and within patient groups. There might be additional funds to remove some of the more glaring holes in health policy through initiatives such as those around reducing waiting lists, but most informed thought saw the need to address the issue of health care rationing explicitly. Unusually, given that health policy is marked by a profound Left/Right divide, it is interesting to note that those most in favour of grasping the rationing nettle do so from a position of defending state-funded health care rather than seeking its replacement. This political location has, in turn, had profound effects on the acceptability of rationing among many who might be thought to be against it on principle.

The case for rationing health services

In recognizing the constraints that the Beveridge fallacy placed on health policy, Thwaites (1987) points out three issues demanding the adoption of a clear position on rationing:

1   increases in the number of older people;
2   the seemingly run-away cost of medical technology;
3   increasing public expectations of what can be provided by a health care system.

In framing the rationing debate these three issues have become something of a mantra among policy analysts. In the following sections we subject them to a brief but critical review.

An ageing population

Demographic change has been highlighted as a crucial component of the crisis in welfare and health care. The spectre of an increasingly ageing population haunts the literature of rationing. Some have interpreted demographic change as a 'generational crisis', with the elderly placing increasing burdens on health care budgets (Thomasma, 1987). This debate has been driven by a perception of older people as 'the elderly' who are a 'burden' in social, economic and health care terms. Indeed, 'the elderly' have, for some time now, been perceived as a 'new social threat' (Callahan, 1987). This analysis has underpinned rationing debates and reinforced views about rationing according to age-based criteria (Williams, 1997). Others, however, have argued that rationing is not an inevitable consequence of an ageing population and that the health care cost crisis is being generated by policy failures. Fries (1980) argues that older people will not necessarily represent a massive burden of chronic illness to society. Instead, there may be a compression of morbidity in later life as the life span, during which functional ability is optimized, is extended. An ageing population does not necessarily lead to cost crisis unless the demographic change is accompanied by a disproportionate growth in the use of health services by older people (Barer et al., 1987). Recent research linking health care expenditure to age suggests that expenditure depends upon remaining lifetime not upon calendar age and that population ageing may not have such a dramatic effect on health care costs as is often assumed (Zweifel et al., 1999). The 'problem' of old age therefore may be a red herring that acts as a convenient justification for cost containment in health and social services spending (Walker, 1995; Phillipson, 1998).

The expansion of technology

The capabilities of medical technology and the increasingly sophistication of clinical techniques have been identified as key factors in increasing demands on health care budgets (Klein et al., 1996;

Stevens *et al.*, 1999). Particular conditions and treatments have become the focus for rationing debates. End-stage renal failure and neo-natal intensive care are two areas where the high cost of treatment has brought particular patient groups into the rationing frame (Mugford, 1988; Jones, 1999). In Britain concerns with the potential cost of prescribed drugs has led to government (and quasi-government) action on drugs for impotence and influenza (Yamey, 1999). In such an environment the fears generated by the orthodox position seem unassailable. However, others have argued that medical technology does not necessarily lead to increasing costs. Cost inflation depends on demand for new technologies and their net effect on the use of other services. It is important to look beyond the spectre of infinite demand perpetuated by politicians and policy makers alike to take a critical view of the reality behind it (Frankel, 1991). Variations in English District Health Authority policies towards in vitro fertilization (IVF) suggest that cost may be a convenient smokescreen for more subjective criteria for rationing services (Redmaynew and Klein, 1993).

An important aspect of the growth of technology is the significance of assessing the opportunity costs related to the introduction of new techniques and products. What benefits and options are created or given up are an essential part of the rational decision-making process. This fuels a demand for reliable and accurate information on the relative effectiveness of treatments and their comparative costs and benefits. This imperative drives the expansion in Evidence Based Health Care (EBHC), which has been institutionalized in organizations such as the National Institute for Clinical Evidence (NICE), which can recommend whether or not treatments should be utilized by the NHS.

This is an important development given that it is linked to fears about expensive new technologies and to evidence suggesting significant levels of publicly funded 'inappropriate', if not harmful, health care (Roos *et al.*, 1990). But as advocates of EBHC themselves have recognized (Chalmers, 1995), EBHC cannot offer certainties. The generalizability of evidence has been questioned while some have interpreted the emphasis on problem solving within the context of randomized controlled trials and meta-analyses as being over-restrictive in focus (Dowie, 1996). The manner in which new technologies are taken up in practice is important, particularly in the way this is mediated by lay–professional relationships. It is here that the apparent certainties that

EBHC produces are subjected to the 'uncertainties' associated with processes of persuasion, decision making, implementation and confirmation. A potential danger lies in the elevation of EBHC by policy makers as a panacea to controlling costs, legitimizing difficult or unpopular decisions and, maybe most importantly, as a way out of the rationing debate. With respect to the expansion of health care technology, the irony that this appears to be met by an expansion in technocratic research should not escape us.

The crisis of expectations

Public support for the NHS remains strong and is mirrored by public support for the welfare state in other European countries. Comparative research has shown that public opinion across Europe supports the prioritization of welfare services to support ageing populations, the need for health care and the need for adequate pensions provision (Taylor-Gooby, 1995). However, this has to be viewed against the context in which the welfare state operates and the aspirations that many in the population have regarding their own standard of living and how the public sector fits in with it. The idea of citizenship as espoused by writers such as T.H. Marshall and Richard Titmuss was one founded on the idea of social rights. These rights would address the fundamental inequalities of a market system by providing the mass of the population with protection against the effects of unemployment, ill health and growing old. The institutions of the welfare state were to provide benefits and services to the mass of the population who either made use of them or knew that they could make use of them.

The establishment of the NHS was conceived very much in this light and, as we have already seen, it was soon subject to conflicts between funding and aspiration. What is interesting is that as other aspects of the welfare state have been transformed (unemployment benefit and social security), rejected (council housing) and marginalized (state retirement pensions), the NHS has retained its popularity (if not necessarily public confidence). One series of arguments as to why this has occurred relates to the role of the welfare state in delivering 'socialized consumption'. In a world where many can participate in privatized consumption and relate this experience to choice, the attractiveness of welfare services and the status of welfare recipient is low. In fact, argues Bauman (1998), to receive services or benefits from the state is a stigmatizing condition separating individuals out from the mass of consumers and locating them as dependent rather than independent. The protection envisaged by the creators of the welfare state that resulted from its mass collective nature is now often seen to be the concern of the few who need the services rather than as being part of the day-to-day reality of the majority. This does not mean that the majority of the population has rejected the welfare state, but rather that it plays less of a role in their lives. Obviously, the minority who are enmeshed in the welfare state experience the reverse of this. The exceptions to this rule – health and education – do play a role in most people's lives either in terms of foreseeable or actual need. This role is, however, also transformed as many of the expectations of consumerism are transferred to these areas in the form of performance leagues, consumer choice and branding.

Consequently, while the ideal of universal and free NHS still appeals because it solves the dilemma of personal and collective risk, it is also put in the position of needing to respond to the transformation of health into an aspect of consumer society. Dealing with disease and disability may have been the main task of a modernist medicine but the issues surrounding the idea of health are much more complex and not just because they have positive rather than negative connotations. The healthy person is also the fit person, who is also the attractive person, who is also the happy person. All aspects of life and the construction of lifestyle are involved in the 'modern imperative of health'. This is not just an individual issue but, as Lupton (1995) among others has pointed out, involves all levels of society including the state. The demands put on health services have not only increased in volume but also in terms of what is expected and how it is delivered. Health care services are expected to be involved, not only in providing for the ill within the hospital and surgery, but also in the community. Through the discourses of public health the population's lifestyles and behaviours are also appropriate arenas for health care involvement. Such 'surveillance medicine', it can be argued, makes each moment of every individual's life, whether they are healthy or sick, a part of health care. In the search for individual health the population expects the health care system to play a role. How each individual defines what is appropriate may differ considerably, but it is noteworthy that many of the most contentious issues regarding demands on health resources have been around 'elective' procedures often involving quality of life or lifestyles. Fertility treatment and the prescription of the drug Viagra for male impotence are two issues from the 1990s that have been subject to resource constraint.

If the scope of what can be provided is now more contentious than ever before, so too is the way that the unspoken power relations of health care have been challenged. The assumption of an unquestioning expert–layperson interaction can no longer be expected. Part of the effect of consumerism and the increase in access to knowledge is the empowerment of the patient. Patients may know what they want and may expect health professionals to deliver it. Dissatisfaction is now monitored and can lead to litigation. How a system such as the NHS can deal with these changes has been one of the motors pushing reform of the role of a publicly funded health care system.

The inevitability of rationing health care?

It would appear from this brief overview that the crises of ageing, technology and expectations are just as much cultural as they are monetary. Indeed, Harrison and Moran (2000) point out that by themselves these 'crises' are insufficient conditions for increasing health care costs. Instead, discussions about demand focus on what is known as 'moral hazard', which is assumed to be prevalent in systems of third-party payment such as the NHS, where the costs of insuring against risk are shared by the whole population (Arrow, 1963). The literature on moral hazard identifies two general forms: provider moral hazard, where providers have an incentive to stimulate demand in order to generate extra revenue; and consumer moral hazard, where consumers are encouraged to increase their demands by not incurring extra costs for extra or new services. For Harrison and Moran the 1990s were marked by a shift towards controlling *demand* through a public discussion of 'inappropriate' use of health services rather than deal with provider-led growth. They add that this shift might only be provisional but it is the balance between demand-side measures and supply-side measures that allows us a clearer understanding of the sources of the rationing debate.

In Britain there are discernible tendencies towards more public discussion of rationing. The acceptance by the English Health

Secretary that rationing is part of the government's modernization of the health services is considered a crucial event (Yamey, 2000), marking a break with the previous reluctance of politicians to mention rationing. The setting up of the NICE forms a 'technocratic' arm to the government's attempts to tackle the problem of rationing health care. While these tendencies have contradictory elements within them, particularly in relation to controlling the pharmaceutical industry, we would argue that the over-arching consensus is illustrated by the references made to the 'given', 'natural' state of rationing.

The shift towards more open debate therefore contains within it a danger of political debate being replaced by the language of prioritization. This can be seen in how lay opinion has been brought into the debate – not as a way of checking the parameters of public acceptance, but rather as something to be brought into line with 'expert' conclusions. Lay knowledge often challenges the authority of professionals to determine the way in which questions are framed, problems are defined and knowledge is used in the policy arena (Williams and Popay, 1994). Dicker and Armstrong (1995), in their study of patients' views of priority setting in health care, found strong support for the principle of equity and collectivist notions of health care. Recurring themes included: lack of acceptance that prioritization should be necessary, belief that doctors should act as the public's advocates and no faith in politicians' views on priorities. Studies of public ranking of different treatments demonstrate different understandings to those of professionals and managers (Bowling, 1993). Some have seen this discrepancy as a product of confusion and argue that public opinions change when they are subjected to systematic debate (Dolan et al., 1999). The role of the media is seen to undermine the possibility of rational debate as public views depend too heavily on media representations of health care dilemmas. For example, Freemantle and Harrison (1993) have identified a tendency among the popular press to present simplistic and one-dimensional views of rationing dilemmas, personalizing what are profound social issues by offering mythical versions of events. However, this is not just a problem of sensationalism confined to the tabloid press, Freemantle and Harrison also identified a technocratic mythology in the so-called quality papers which was based on de-personalizing rationing dilemmas and turning them into technical issues. In this alternative mythology vociferous patient groups and popular campaigns over resources are presented as 'problematic' rather than related to notions of citizenship and rights.

In the light of the evidence presented above which suggests an inexorable drift towards both rationing and a public debate on its acceptability, what can sociology in general, and a Habermas-influenced critical theory in particular, say about the phenomenon? More importantly, are we now facing an acceptance of the limitation of the universalism of the NHS, as many of the proponents of the necessity for rationing would hope, or is there still profound conflict rather than consensus? The justification for accepting rationing hinges on the acceptance that it represents a rational response to changing circumstances. Such rationality seems neutral and feeds into the idea of the rationalization of the welfare state. We would argue that the conclusions reached represent only a particular form of rationality – one that mini-mizes the importance of different starting points and a different rationality. Consequently, calls to limit health care by rationing cannot be divorced from wider social processes and interests. For example, evidence of increasing inequalities in health (Gordon *et al*., 1999) should raise concerns about the burden of costs being unfairly placed on the most vulnerable in society. If calls for public debates of rationing are prefaced by 'rational' parameters framed by pre-existing discourses, we need to address what we mean by rationality and rationalization.

Rationality and rationalization

As is well known, it is the work of Max Weber that is most iden-tified with describing the institutionalization of scientific and technical rationality in the development of modern western soci-eties (Weber, 1979). A major feature of this work was an examination of the extension of scientific and technological deci-sion making into the different areas of social life previously governed by traditional social organization and values (Giddens, 1971). This development was seen as an inevitable consequence of industrialization and modernity and was encapsulated in the notion of the 'iron cage of rationalisation' which described an arena of purposive-rationality where human action was severely limited. The fatalistic and pessimistic consequences of this posi-tion in Weber's work are well known (Turner, 1993) and have been very influential. It is a theme present in the work of the Frankfurt School (Turner, 1996) and even in the Marxism of Georg Lukács (Lowy, 1979). What emerges from Weber is a belief that rationalization and rationalized systems led to a diminution of human subjectivity and that this was the inevitable nature of modern life.

The work of Habermas needs to be placed in this context if we are to use it to throw light on the questions surrounding rationing of health services and the way the public is being brought into the debate. Habermas believes that while many of the things Weber wrote concerning rationalization are valuable, he was wrong in ascribing primacy to the rationalization of structures of power over culture and ethics. Weber pays insufficient attention to the rationalization of ethics and culture which, Habermas asserts, are equally involved in the development of rationalized society through setting limits to what can and cannot be regarded as legitimate. These limits act as a brake on power and have the ability to create demands on society out of their own 'inner logic'. By doing this Habermas breaks out of the fatalism and pessimism of the 'iron cage'. The distinction Habermas makes between 'purposive rational action' and 'communicative action' helps us to understand this. Following from his discussion of the rationalization process, purposive-rational action is analogous to Weber's *Zweckrationalitat* while communicative action is a form of linguistic interaction aimed at achieving understanding founded on shared values. These two processes form the basis of what Habermas describes in turn as the system-world and the lifeworld. The system-world is involved in the distribution of power and resources while the lifeworld is concerned with the reproduction of values and culture.

In this formulation it is important to note that these two worlds are not in balance but are connected by the continuing dialectic between culture and structure in which structure presently grossly overwhelms culture. Developing themes implicit in 'Critical Theory' Habermas follows Marcuse in suggesting that rationality can itself be a form of domination of social relations as purposive-rational action follows the dictates of power and becomes an exercise in control rather than a product of common values. What then occurs is the replacement of the beneficial aspects of rationalization with those that lead to domination.

Accordingly, Habermas argues that the late twentieth century has seen a move away from the 'art' of administration (as envisaged by Weber) to a new scientific stage of bureaucratization.

> The scientization of politics is not yet a reality, but it is a real tendency for which there is evidence.
>
> (Habermas, 1989: 62)

Instead of Weber's distinction between the expert (working in technical and scientific spaces) and the politician (working in space characterized by the operation of power and the will), in the new scientific stage this division becomes blurred. To account for these changes Habermas outlines three models of bureaucratization:

The Technocratic model – where the politician is now dependent on and is an agent of a scientific intelligentsia.

The Expanded decisionistic model – where new technocrats camouflage what is as political as ever (although it is now constrained by technocratic rules).

The Pragmatic model – involving critical interaction between expert and politician in a loop of communicative practice.

Following from our discussion of health care rationing in Britain it is possible to discern technocratic and decisionistic tendencies in current debates. Indeed, one of the enduring characteristics of the debate regarding rationing is that of experts bemoaning the public's susceptibility to 'shroud waving' and constructing more and more abstract ways to make priority setting as technical and value free as possible. The notion that the public might not accept any such limits is increasingly constrained by their seeming irrationality. However, Habermas does not accept the pessimistic view that there is a necessary triumph of bureaucratic rationalization. The equal development of ethical rationalization also means other issues such as values and democracy must be addressed. Habermas certainly sees tensions between democracy and technocratic administration because the latter's objective status and axiomatic role make political will (be it that of political elites or of the people) increasingly redundant.

The de-politicization of the mass of the population and the decline of the public realm as a political institution are components of a system of domination that tends to exclude practical questions from public discussion. The bureaucratized exercise of power has its counterpart in a public realm confined to spectacles and acclamation.

(Habermas, 1989: 75)

Modern secular societies are increasingly characterized as internally differentiated and pluralized. In such circumstances Habermas argues that validity (that is, rationally motivated beliefs) and facticity (that is, the force of external sanctions based on fact) become incompatible (Habermas, 1996). The answer for Habermas lies with a deliberative democracy where a discursive model of the law (based on communicative practices) replaces a contractual model. At the heart of his argument is the view that there is an internal relation between the rule of law and democracy. This means that the rule of law is contingent on radical democracy:

... private legal subjects cannot come to enjoy equal individual liberties if they do not *themselves*, in the common exercise of their political autonomy, achieve clarity about justified interests and standards. They themselves must agree on the relevant aspects under which equals should be treated equally and unequals unequally.

(Habermas, 1996: xlii; original emphasis)

How this is to be done and whether or not it is achievable is probably the most difficult set of tasks. How is agreement on equal treatment to be made compatible with the structured inequality of power in society?

From philosophy to policy

Len Doyal (1995, 1997) has most notably tried to lay down broad principles for decision making derived from the work of Habermas. Drawing on work he wrote with Ian Gough (Doyal and Gough, 1991), he has emphasized the importance both of physiological needs and the need for autonomy in any decision making. In contrast to a number of writers who argue for implicit decision making (Coast, 1997; Hunter, 1995), Doyal argues that all decision making must be done explicitly if it is going to be fair.

The view that rationing must be made explicit is in line with the Habermasian notion of publicly accountable speech acts and presents us with an *optimistic* approach to issues of policy implementation. This optimism is founded on the assumption that there are possibilities of agreement over normative judgements in the allocation of resources. This is not to say that such agreement exists as of now. Rather, it is to say that this is the best principle on which to base policy, recognizing that the processes and outcomes of policy are always imperfect. The notion that implicit rationing is preferable can be seen as a *pessimistic* response to the issues of policy making by implying that there can be no real debate on prioritization that doesn't become unfair for one group or another. In contradistinction it allows decision making to become an assemblage of individual decisions that create gaps in overall policies for some localized benefit to occur to particular groups.

Both camps accordingly accept prioritization as a principle for the allocation of resources, the argument between them concerns how this should be done and by whom. Many would reject implicit methods of rationing because such an approach denies any possibility of debate and might even hide the assumptions on which powerful groups base their decisions. However, explicit discussion of resource allocation decisions has the potential to create similar outcomes. Agreement about the relevant aspects of health care where equals are treated equally and unequals are treated unequally is always vulnerable to distortion through the colonization of the lifeworld by medicine (Scambler, 1987). Such colonization has occurred through the social respect attributed to medical expertise, its social legitimation, and its formal knowledge (Friedson, 1986). This is not to say that such colonization has only one dimension. The positive aspect of medicine is in the contribution it makes to the meeting of generalizable needs and interests. Unfortunately, these are combined with the negative aspects of social control found in the inappropriate use of formal medical knowledge to justify or legitimate the vested interests of the powerful. It is here that we believe the problem of ideology has to be re-addressed given the way that all decisions are embrocated in structured power. The rejection by many of the legitimacy of rationing health care is an example of such an awareness; an awareness that limits to resources are only partial and not extended to those whose wealth can buy a way out.

Ideology

It seems to us that the real issues surrounding ideology are insufficiently addressed in discussions of rationing. This is not because it is not recognized as an important issue; rather, it is because the use of the term is shorthand for politics. For example, Sir John Grimley-Evans makes the following point in constructing an argument against age-based rationing:

> I am convinced that in the UK at present it is unethical to use age as a criterion for depriving people of health care from which they could benefit. The fundamental issue is ideological; and ideologies – and the ethical systems derived from them – can change with circumstances.
>
> (Grimley-Evans, 1997)

While the point is correct, leaving the idea of ideology at this level does little more than tell us that people with different points of view see things differently. The concept of ideology can offer us much more if it is used in systematic and appropriate ways. We are aware that the whole issue of ideology is one that is embroiled in numerous disputes about terminology and context (see for example Eagleton, 1991 or Larrain, 1979). We have no desire to join this debate, instead, we will use the term to designate ideas, discourses and practices that systematically represent the social world to the benefit of a dominant class.

Using this formulation it is possible to see how the ideas, discourses and practices of those advocating rationing health services can be seen as operating in the realm of ideology. The idea of limited resources is one which when applied to the social rather than the natural world is about choices between competing calls on money within the economic system. Limitations and expansions are driven by social and political contexts. Accepting limits as natural is an ideological assumption. Taking an 'agnostic stance' towards the availability of resources as many health economists would claim is not a neutral position, rather it is one that has no critical dimension.

The discourses surrounding rationing posit it as rational, but once again we would argue that it is a particular form of rationality that is being addressed – an instrumental rationality. Once the assumptions have been accepted then only certain conclusions can be reached even if these conclusions seem less desirable than some of the advocates would want. The discourses of rationing can provide a technocratic legitimacy to shifts in power relations while claiming to be neutral or in fact trying to right particular inequities.

A similar thing can be seen in relation to the practices that emerge from the rationing debates, namely those concerned with democratizing the process and trying to initiate a public debate. As we have seen, asking the public or trying to involve professional health care workers in the process of prioritization is not so much about finding out what they think but rather 'educating' and 'interpreting' their views. Again, these practices are constituted as ideological practices because participation is 'bounded' by the practices of a dominant class and the economic system of capitalism.

How does our utilization of the concept of ideology fit with the use of a Habermasian critical theory? We are aware that the term is not used much by Habermas, who sees it as too unreconstructed a Marxist notion. However, we would argue that accepting a colonization of the lifeworld by the system-world demands more of a response than claiming that it is illegitimate. Claiming that the decline of the public sphere is a consequence of media trivialization ignores issues that have received much sociological attention, such as changes towards consumerism and lifestyle. It needs to be connected to an analysis of the ideology of privatism (Harris, 1999). The debate about rationing is about changes in the nature of the postwar welfare state and the role of the citizen. Technocratic discourses seek to create a 'bounded' citizen who is aware that it is his or her responsibility to prosper and make minimal demands on the state. The keywords in this contract are responsibility, efficiency and consultation. The rationing debate provides all of these in abundance. The promise of efficiency and participation are falsehoods for all the reasons Habermas has outlined in his work on system- and lifeworlds and on deliberative democracy. The only values that are accepted are those belonging to the system-world and the only deliberation possible is that of accepting them.

As a consequence of this we would suggest that those aspects of Habermas' work which relate most to his attachment to historical materialism need to be revisited. The issue of ideology that we have brought up is one that causes difficulty as far as many critical theorists are concerned (Bohman, 1999). The utilization of the term ideology suggests a more determinate relationship between understanding and social structure than one of critiquing assumptions as in much critical theory. We do not have space to take this argument further but we raise it as a point for consideration, particularly if we are to address the idea of human emancipation.

Conclusion

The struggle between technocratic and popular approaches to the issue of rationing health care is ultimately a political conflict. Behind the difficult terminology of Habermas' approach to rationality and modernity is the familiar terrain of Left and Right and, more significantly, the ever-present resistance to the partial concerns of the powerful. The reluctance of large parts of the population to countenance rationing health care is the product of a de-commodified position on which the lifeworld is based. The technocratic appeal to finite resources is an acceptance of limitations imposed on health care by system rationality. It is not likely that there will be a resolution of this contradiction over time given the very different starting points involved. It may be the case, as the welfare state changes, that some of the concerns of technocratic rationality start to permeate the lifeworld as the campaign to accept limited financial resources centres on what constitutes a legitimate starting point. To return for a moment to the problem of age-based rationing, two works by Habermas-influenced policy analysts (Longino and Murphy, 1995; Moody, 1995) accept the need to reduce health expenditures on older people in order that a more humanistic health policy can emerge. The former argue that biomedicine fails older people by concentrating on high-tech interventions that are inappropriate to their needs and go on to give guarded support to the Oregon Plan as a flawed attempt to collectively decide health resources. Moody on the other hand sees terrible consequences for all in an ageing population and advocates setting limits to life so that the lifeworld can regain control over old age. It would seem, that as Albrow (1987) has pointed out, the system-world itself generates a value system, and this may become a basis for general social values.

In conclusion, the issue of rationing health care is an example of the contradictions that exist in the modern world between very different models of social organization. We have used the work of Habermas to describe and account for this divide, but it may be that the abstract distinction between system- and lifeworld can only provide us with the starting point for an analysis of the relations between society, technocrats and health care rationing. More importantly we have shown that the concept of class-based ideology is crucial to understanding why the conflicts over rationing are more fundamental than disputes about rationality. If we have achieved anything in this chapter it is drawing attention to this omission from the mainstream debate.

References

Albrow, M. (1987) 'The application of the Weberian concept of rationalisation to contemporary conditions'. In Whimster, S. and Lash, S. (eds) *Max Weber, Rationality and Modernity*. London: Allen & Unwin.

Annandale, E. (1998) *The Sociology of Health and Medicine: A Critical Introduction*. Cambridge: Polity Press.

Arrow, K. (1963) 'Uncertainty and the welfare economics of medical care'. *American Economic Review*, 53: 941–73.

Barer, M.L., Evans, R.G., Hetzman, C. and Lomas, J. (1987) 'Ageing and health care utilization: new evidence on old fallacies'. *Social Science and Medicine*, 24, 10: 852–62.

Bauman, Z. (1998) *Work, Consumerism and the New Poor*. Buckingham: Open University Press.

Bohman, J. (1999) 'Habermas, Marxism and Social Theory: the case for pluralism in critical social science'. In Dews, P. (ed.) *Habermas: A Critical Reader*. Oxford: Blackwell.

Bowling, A. (1993) *What People Say About Prioritising Health Services*. London: King's Fund Centre.

Callahan, D. (1987) *Setting Limits: Medical Goals in an Ageing Society*. New York: Simon & Schuster.

Chalmers, I. (1995) 'Letter, What would Archie Cochrane have said?' *Lancet*, 346: 1300.

Coast, J. (1997) 'The rationing debate: rationing within the NHS should be explicit: the case against'. *British Medical Journal*, 314: 1118.

Dicker, A, and Armstrong, D. (1995) 'Patients' views of priority setting in health care: an interview survey in one practice'. *British Medical Journal*, 311: 1137–9.

Dolan, P., Cookson, R. and Ferguson, B. (1999) 'Effect of discussion and deliberation on the public's views of priority setting in health care: focus group study'. *British Medical Journal*, 318: 916–19.

Dowie, J. (1996) 'The research practice gap and the role of decision analysis in closing it'. *Health Care Analysis*, 4, 1: 5–18.

Doyal, L. (1995) 'Needs, rights, and equity: moral quality in health care rationing'. *Quality in Health Care*, 4: 273–83.

—— (1997) 'The rationing debate: rationing within the NHS should be explicit: the case for'. *British Medical Journal*, 314: 1114.

Doyal, L. and Gough, I. (1991) *A Theory of Human Need*. London: Macmillan.

Eagleton, T. (1991) *Ideology*. London: Verso.

Frankel, S. (1991) 'Health needs, health care requirements and the myth of infinite demand'. *Lancet*, 337: 1588–9.

Freemantle, N. and Harrison, S. (1993) 'Interlukin-2: the public and professional face of rationing in the NHS'. *Critical Social Policy*, 37: 94–117.

Friedson, E. (1986) *Professional Powers: A Study of the Institutionalisation of Formal Knowledge*. Chicago, IL: University of Chicago Press.

Fries, J. (1980) 'Ageing, natural death and the compression of morbidity'. *New England Journal of Medicine*, 303, 13: 130.

Giddens, A. (1971) *Capitalism and Modern Social Theory*. Cambridge: Cambridge University Press.

Gordon, D., Shaw, M., Dorling, D. and Smith, G.D. (eds) (1999) *Inequalities in Health: The Evidence Presented to the Independent Inquiry into Inequalities in Health, Chaired by Sir Donald Acheson*. Bristol: Policy Press.

Grimley-Evans, J. (1997) 'Rationing health care by age: the case against'. In New, B. (ed.) *Rationing Talk and Action*. London: British Medical Journal publishing group.

Habermas, J. (1989) *Towards a Rational Society*. Cambridge: Polity Press.

—— (1996) *Between Facts and Norms: Contributors to a Discourse Theory of Law and Democracy*. Cambridge, MA: MIT Press.

Harris, J. (1999) 'State social work and social citizenship in Britain: from clientelism to consumerism'. *British Journal of Social Work*, 29: 915–37.

Harrison, S. and Moran, M. (2000) 'Resources and rationing: managing supply and demand in health care'. In Albrecht, G.L., Fitzpatrick, R. and Scrimshaw, S.C. (eds) *The Handbook of Social Studies in Health and Medicine*. London: Sage.

Higgs, P. (1993) *The NHS and Ideological Conflict*. Aldershot: Avebury.

Hunter, D.J. (1995) 'Rationing health care: the political perspective'. *British Medical Bulletin*, 51, 4: 876–84.

Jones, I.R. (1999) *Professional Power and the Need for Health Care*. Aldershot: Ashgate.

Klein, R. (1991) 'On the Oregon Trail: rationing health care' (Editorial). *British Medical Journal*, 302, 6767: 1–2.

Klein, R.E., Day, P. and Redmayne, S. (1996) *Priority Setting and Rationing in the National Health Service*. Buckingham: Open University Press.

Larrain, J. (1979) *The Concept of Ideology*. London: Hutchinson.

Longino, C. and Murphy, J. (1995) *The Old Age Challenge to the Biomedical Model: Paradigm Strain and Health Policy*. Amityville: Baywood.

Lowy, M. (1979) *Georg Lukács – From Romantic to Revolutionary*. London: New Left Books.

Lupton, D. (1995) *The Imperative of Health*. London: Sage.

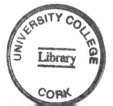

Moody, H. (1995) 'Ageing, meaning and the allocation of resources'. *Ageing and Society*, 15: 163–84.

Mugford, M. (1988) 'A review of the economics of care of sick new born infants'. *Community Medicine*, 10, 2: 99–111.

New, B. (1996) 'The rationing agenda in the NHS'. *British Medical Journal*, 312: 1593–1601.

Phillipson, C. (1998) *Reconstructing Old Age*. London: Sage.

Redmaynew, S. and Klein, R. (1993) 'Rationing in practice: the case of in vitro fertilisation'. *British Medical Journal*, 306: 1521–4.

Roos, L.L., Brazouskas, R., Cohen, M.M. and Sharp, S.M. (1990) 'Variations in outcome research'. In Anderson, T.F. and Mooney, G. (eds) *The Challenges of Medical Practice Variations*. Basingstoke: Macmillan Press.

Scambler, G. (1987) 'Habermas and the power of medical expertise'. In Scambler, G. (ed.) *Sociological Theory and Medical Sociology*. London: Tavistock.

Stevens, A., Milne, R., Lilford, R. and Gabbay, J. (1999) 'Keeping pace with new technologies: systems needed to identify and evaluate them'. *British Medical Journal*, 319: 1291.

Taylor-Gooby, P. (1995) 'Who wants the welfare state? Support for state welfare in European countries.' In Svallfors, S. (ed.) *In the Eye of the Beholder*. Umea, Sweden: Impello Saljsupport.

Thomasma, D.C. (1987) 'Moving the aged into the house of the dead'. *Journal of the American Geriatrics Society*, 37, 2: 169–72.

Thwaites, B. (1987) *The NHS: The End of the Rainbow? The Foundation Lecture*. Southampton: Institute of Health Policy Studies, University of Southampton.

Turner, B. (1993) *Max Weber: From History to Modernity*. London: Routledge.

—— (1996) *For Weber: Essays on the Sociology of Fate*. London: Sage.

Walker, A. (1995) *Half a Century of Promises*. London: Counsel and Care.

Weber, M. (1979) *Economy and Society*. Berkeley: University of California Press.

Williams, A. (1997) 'The rationing debate: rationing health care by age: the case for'. *British Medical Journal*, 314: 820–2.

Williams, G. and Popay, J. (1994) 'Researching the people's health: dilemmas and opportunities for social scientists'. In Popay, J. and Williams, G. (eds) *Researching the People's Health*. London: Routledge.

Yamey, G. (1999) 'Dobson backed NICE ruling on flu drug'. *British Medical Journal*, 319: 1024.

—— (2000) 'Health secretary admits that NHS rationing is government policy'. *British Medical Journal*, 320: 10.

Zweifel, P., Felder, S. and Meiers, M. (1999) 'Ageing of population and health care expenditure: a red herring?' *Health Economics*, 8: 485–96.

Chapter 8

Habermas or Foucault or Habermas and Foucault?

The implications of a shifting debate for medical sociology

Ian Rees Jones

I call interactions *communicative* when the participants co-ordinate their plans of action consensually, with the agreement reached at any point being evaluated in terms of the intersubjective recognition of validity claims. In cases where agreement is reached through explicit linguistic processes, the actors make three different claims to validity in their speech acts as they come to agreement with one another about something. Those claims are claims to truth, claims to rightness, and claims to truthfulness, according to whether the speaker refers to something in the objective world (as the totality of existing states of affairs), to something in the shared world (as the totality of the legitimately regulated interpersonal relationships of a social group), or to something in his own subjective world (as the totality of experiences to which one has privileged access).

(Habermas, 1990: 58)

In the serious play of questions and answers, in the work of reciprocal elucidation, the rights of each person are in some sense immanent in the discussion. They depend only on the dialogue situation. The person asking the questions is merely exercising the right that has been given him: to remain unconvinced, to perceive contradiction, to require more information, to emphasize different postulates, to point out faulty reasoning, etc. As for the person answering the questions, he too exercises a right that does not go beyond the discussion itself; by the logic of his own discourse he is tied to what he has said earlier, and by the acceptance of dialogue he is tied to the questioning of the other. Questions and answers depend on a game – a game that is at once pleasant and difficult – in which each of

the two partners takes pains to use only the rights given him by
the other and by the accepted form of the dialogue.

(Foucault, 1984: 381)

Introduction

The quotations from Habermas and Foucault seem to me to
highlight the tensions, contradictions and correspondences in their
work. Michael Kelly reminds us that the question of universals such
as 'truth' is at the heart of the Foucault/Habermas debate, but our
understanding of this is not helped by casting their arguments in
'relativist versus absolutist' terms (Kelly, 1994). Thomas McCarthy
(1994) has argued that Foucault and the Frankfurt School are more
closely related than the froth of argument and disagreement
between their disciples would suggest. He argues that the strengths
of Foucault's oeuvre can be used to complement critical theory so
that rather than choosing between them we should strive to
'combine them in constructing theoretically informed and
practically interested histories of the present' (McCarthy, 1994:
273). This chapter will explore the possibilities of such an approach
for sociological understandings of health and health care. It has
become common to distinguish between the early and later
Foucault, with some writers suggesting that the later Foucault was
working towards ways of addressing the criticisms of his earlier
work through the construction of an ethics of care. Others have
cautioned against reading too much into what is unfinished work,
maintaining that although he was moving in new directions it would
be overstating the case to describe the differences between his earlier
and later work as a rupture. It is also becoming increasingly
common to distinguish between Habermas' concern with communicative practices and more recent work from the beginning of the
1990s onwards which has focused on justice and norms in political
democracy. Medical sociologists have used the work of both writers
to expose the irony in the vain attempts by some policy makers,
public health practitioners, clinicians, managers and politicians to
neutralize the politics of health by cloaking it in 'value free' technocratic procedures. Some writers have started to examine the later
works of both writers, seeing in both the stimulus for attempts to
address the political paralysis and conservatism that appear to be at
the heart of the postmodern dilemma. By focusing on Foucault's
later work and Habermas' more recent concerns, my aim in this

chapter is to speculate on the ways in which the work of both writers can illuminate our understandings of areas that are of key concern to the sociology of health and illness at this point in time. I will begin by outlining the Foucault/Habermas debate, focusing on their approaches to modernity, power and truth, before considering the interactions between their later work. I will consider the relevance of Foucault and Habermas in relation to three key areas: changes in our understanding of medicalization, the consequences of globalization for health and health care and the increasing relevance of surveillance and governmentality.

Power, truth and acting subjects

Habermas has occupied himself with attempting to rescue the enlightenment project from what has been termed its dialectic; that is, in the face of its promised freedoms based on progress, modernity also produced fear, censorship and repression. Foucault addresses this dialectic through a historicity or genealogy of reason. Habermas addresses it by attempting to define what reason *really* is. The problem of modernity for Foucault is that it is doomed once knowledge becomes reflective whereas Habermas finds modernity's emancipatory dimension dormant. Habermas' communicative procedures are the means by which discourse can enable emancipation. Foucault however suggests that discourse captures and then signifies the death of subject. The challenge to Habermas' attempt to rescue the enlightenment project by means of a theory of communicative rationality comes from Foucault's dismissal of negative interpretations of power. The problem becomes one of distinguishing between different types of rationality when, as Foucault argues, the effects of power may be all pervasive and truth is contingent and a thing of this world (Foucault, 1984). When stated in these terms it is difficult to see the correspondences between these two writers. To begin to do so it is necessary to consider their approaches to power and truth in more depth.

Power

Foucault sees power as a creative force that by virtue of 'multiple forms of constraint' is an inherent part of the production of truth (Foucault, 1980). This allows him to argue that medical practitioners have been able to classify, observe and experiment on the bodies of subjects by means of a set of power relations that provide the means to further knowledge. At the same time these power relations allow the medical profession to take that knowledge into judicial spheres to legitimize their claim to expand their areas of practice (Philip, 1990). Through a multiplicity of such power relations, operating through institutions and human sciences (asylums and medical knowledge being popular examples), power saturates the social field. Foucault emphasized the way disciplinary power subjects bodies to normalization through what he termed 'biopower'. The important point here is that biopower is deemed to be immune to critical discourse. Any attempt to disentangle legitimate and illegitimate facets to biopower runs the danger of reinforcing the violent effects of normalization on the body.

Foucault's critique of power, however, can only be constructed by reference to normative notions (Fraser, 1989). Habermas has argued that Foucault ignored the development of normative structures in connection with the modern formation of power (Habermas, 1992). As Giddens points out, Foucault leaves little room for the concept of agency or the individual embodying it (Giddens, 1982). Habermas' critique of Foucault sees his genealogies caught in a performative contradiction in that, when part of the critique requires putting all claims of validity in doubt, why accept this critique as any more valid than others? Put simply, if critique is a form of power then Foucault contradicts himself because it cannot then be used to criticize power. Foucault's concept of power makes it impossible for any analysis to distinguish between different degrees of power and obscures the structural origins of differences in power in social relations (Porter, 1996). If power is everywhere my saying no to my son's request for more ice cream or telling my daughter that she must go to school today are indistinguishable from the operation of power in the bombing of Kosovo. Some would take issue with my choice of comparisons (perhaps saying all they reveal are an ingrained sense of Calvinistic Puritanism) but at a deeper level Hoy (1998), for example, argues that the argument of performative contradiction misunderstands Foucault's position, which is to make the familiar unfamiliar. He suggests that genealogy is a way of diagnosing asymmetries of power that are derived from scientific knowledge. White (1997) argues in similar vein that Foucault held a relational concept of power and that this needs to be distinguished from notions of repression or domination. These arguments, however, seem to equate Foucault's genealogy with sociological method. Habermas' processes of communication are in one sense an attempt to neutralize the negative effects of domination and power. Foucault interprets power as having both negative and positive effects, thus suggesting that any attempt to neutralize these involves absolute forms of judgement. In this sense Habermas is seemingly accused of a conceit. Foucault's relativism, however, leaves him open to the charge of political impotence. His response to the problem of resistance to oppressive forces was not always consistent but in his later work he seems to accept that the means to minimize the effects of domination are to be found in legal rules as well as in the practices of self (Hoy, 1998). Unfortunately it is not clear what form these legal rules might take.

Truth

Foucault utilizes a rhetoric in his writing that is deliberatively disruptive, forcing us to question our understanding of key concepts such as power, truth and freedom. In this way he exposes any attempt to discuss the truth about ourselves as the construction of a specific new discourse that contains within itself new constraints and controls:

> Each society has its own regime of truth, its 'general politics' of truth: that is, the types of discourse which it accepts and makes function as true; the mechanisms and instances which enable one to distinguish true and false statements, the means by which each is sanctioned; the techniques and procedures accorded of those who are charged with stating what counts as true.
>
> (Foucault, 1984: 73).

Foucault argues that the political economy of truth is centred in the form of scientific discourse, is subject to constraint and economic and political incitement, is also the object of immense diffusion and consumption and is produced and transmitted under the control of dominant apparatus. In this sense it is the focus of ideological struggles. He seems to suggest that our concern should not be about discovering truth but uncovering and challenging the accepted rules according to which the true and the false are separated. Foucault therefore sees truth as a system of procedures for the production and distribution of statements linked with systems of power – a 'regime of truth'. The role of the intellectual in the face of this regime is to look for a new politics of truth, not by changing people's minds but by changing the regime of truth where truth is detached from existing hegemonies.

In contrast, Habermas distinguishes between three forms of truth. In the first form he identifies claims of truth that relate to facts and objects that are part of the objective world. In the second form, he identifies claims of rightness that concern the shared world of intersubjective communication. In the third form, he distinguishes claims of truthfulness that are part of the individual subjective world of experience and meaning. Communicative practices are a necessary basis for all three forms. This is because communication would be impossible if our life experiences were completely alien to one another and unnecessary if they corresponded exactly (Bhaskar, 1998). Claims to truth or rightness can be supported by recourse to argumentation and explanation and claims to truthfulness supported by consistent behaviour. It is here that we find a wide gulf between the two writers, as Foucault seems to see demons in discursive acts while Habermas seems to place the communicative process on a philosophical pedestal.

Foucault and the acting subject

Whereas the early Foucault was concerned with forms of state discipline and surveillance, which appeared to deny subjectivity, the later Foucault is specifically concerned with an active subject and with the creative potential of the subject. Here bodies and subjects become not only sites for the gaze of surveillance to wander over but also sites of resistance to power. In seeing power as something that saturated the social field, Foucault's earlier work suggested both a denial of human agency and a futility of protest and resistance. The emphasis he places in his later work on the care of the self seems to be the beginnings of an attempt to break out of this trap (Foucault, 1990). Foucault focuses on the creative potential of an aesthetics of self focused on the body and on texts. He does not relinquish his criticism of normativity (he still insists that there is no *true* self) but the possibilities of an aesthetics of existence are to be found in the *conscious creation* of a self.

It is questionable how this subversion of texts coupled with a focus on the technologies of the self (albeit openly performed) can lead to radical social action. Smart (1998) develops a critique of this emphasis on the care of the self by arguing that Foucault leaves little room for a self that develops through interaction with others. In other words, Foucault's ethics of care privileges the self, because in order to care for others one first of all has to have competency. Smart on the other hand sees care for others as ontological; the two are inseparable and bound by the notion of reciprocity. It is this reciprocity that is at the heart of Habermas' communicative theory and his critique of Foucault (Habermas, 1985). It seems to me that the contrast between Foucault and Habermas is at its deepest here because Foucault's work is based on an impoverished view of social relations and reciprocity.

Habermas and discursive democracy

In his more recent work Habermas has extended the work set out in the theory of communicative action in the direction of democratic institutions and law (Habermas, 1992). This has led to a shift from a focus on the seemingly dualistic concerns of instrumental and communicative rationality, lifeworld and system-world, to a focus on *mediation* (Delanty, 1999). In doing so Habermas seems to be defending a cosmopolitan notion of modernity, in contrast to his earlier writings which were concerned with the enlightenment project. This shift is discernible in his attempt to develop a critique of European democracy (Habermas, 1999). Here Habermas develops the idea of a *discursive democracy* in contrast to both liberal democracy based on constitutional majorities *and* democracy derived from notions of civic community. The pluralistic, multicultural and cosmopolitan features of modern societies demand a different form of democracy based on discursive practices. This is related to Habermas' view that a radical democratic politics is concerned with the extent to which changes in law and institutions can be achieved through and in discursive practices. This seems to suggest democratic institutions need to develop liminal qualities. If discursive democracy is based on universal procedures rather than universal values, it demands both public discussion and protest in the civic public sphere. It is through this prior public argumentation (in various forms) that opinion can be integrated into law and institutional frameworks. In this respect liminality can be interpreted as the capacity of institutional frameworks to change without being destroyed. Lifeworld problems and solutions need to be brought to the surface in the public sphere but solutions can only be implemented in and through the law and institutional processes. This development in Habermas' work seems to address earlier critiques of his concept of the public sphere. It is no longer the rather romanticized notion of a bourgeois public sphere largely separate from the private sphere but now appears as a space where the communication of public opinion is part of a public/private sphere network where differences and argumentation between experts are shaped by public views. The importance of law for Habermas is that it becomes the medium by which lifeworld and system-world are linked. Thus he dismisses the view that the law is a tool of the system of domination as a form of naïve oppositional politics. Delanty (1999) considers this shift to be an important and positive development in Habermas' work but notes that there is still a lack of emphasis on culture, particularly cultural conflict and identity. This weakens Habermas' position in two ways. In the first instance, because cultural conflicts are *endemic* to the lifeworld, the notion of communicative procedure as the basis for conflict resolution seems closer to the discourses of the courtroom and the academic seminar than to the conflicts of deeply divided societies. Is it reasonable to expect individuals and groups to step outside their culture and identities to engage in rational debate? In the second place, while Habermas recognizes that discursive democracy has to operate at a global level, his conception of it seems unable to address the problems associated with a world characterized by global capitalism and a multiplicity of cultural identities. What kind of transnational institutions can address this challenge? Habermas' model is always vulnerable to the critique that he is adopting a Eurocentric approach to the problem of global democracy.

Medicalization, globalization and governmentality

There is insufficient space to consider the breadth of work that is covered by sociologies of and sociologies in medicine and it would be foolhardy to attempt to do so even if there were space. Instead this section will consider three fields where I think the Habermas/Foucault debate has particular relevance. To begin I will consider changes in our understanding of medicalization that are ongoing as a consequence of advances in medical science and technology. I will then look briefly at the implications of globalization for our understanding of health. Finally I will consider the importance of governmentality as an explanatory concept in the field of public health policy.

Medicalization

The success of medical science and technology is heralded every day in newspapers and television. Advances in the new genetics, transplant medicine and cybertechnology are held up as evidence of the dawn of a new age of medical progress. Conrad (1999) has suggested that much of this reporting overstates the case for medical progress and often ignores or downplays cases of negative findings (that is, scientific research that places doubt on the claims being made for these new technologies). At the same time the same media are reporting the problems, fears and anxieties associated with these advances, often in lurid and sensational terms. Medical sociology has a tradition of researching the unease and sense of crisis that is associated with such medical advances. Starting from Illich's (1976) interconnected typologies of iatrogenesis it is possible to trace a line through Friedson's (1986) accounts of medicine in relation to capitalism to recent accounts of globalization and public policy (Reinicke, 1998). It is timely therefore to ask, has our understanding of medicalization changed in recent years and to what extent is this related to shifts in our understanding of truth and power?

Post-structuralist and postmodern accounts have presented a profound challenge to the intellectual roots of medical sociology (Bury, 1997). Followers of these approaches have portrayed health and illness in terms of fragmented and pluralistic practices embedded in discourse. This cultural and linguistic turn has led to a flowering of work, much of which draws on Foucauldian thought. David Armstrong (1994) has produced an impressive body of work based on Foucault (particularly the early Foucault). He has used Foucault's attacks on Whig notions of history and on history in general to develop a critique of medical science and knowledge and humanist notions of medical progress. The foundation of his critique (if it can be described as a foundation) is a strong social constructivism. Foucault's emphasis on the productive nature of power is taken a step further in the hands of strong social constructionists who argue that there is no real human body to be discovered. The 'body' is constructed by and through the prevailing medical gaze. This is perhaps most notably encapsulated in Armstrong's view that 'A body analysed for humours contains humours; a body analysed for organs and tissues is constituted by organs and tissues; a body analysed for psychosocial functioning is a psychosocial object' (Armstrong, 1994: 25). Others have taken similar approaches to critique the breadth of medical involvement in society from dentistry (Nettleton, 1989) to public health (Peterson, 1997).

Deborah Lupton (1994, 1995) has highlighted increasing societal concerns with 'health' and the problems that this open-ended and multifarious concept presents for public health policy and practice. She has also drawn attention to some of the limitations of post-structuralist accounts of health. While criticizing 'orthodox' accounts of medicalization and outlining the advantages of Foucauldian approaches to medicine, she notes that basing a sociology of medicine on Foucauldian lines (particularly the tendency to portray people as 'passive bodies') misses the ways in which lay people interact with medical discourses (Lupton, 1997). Giddens (1992) has used the example of sex addiction to show how the medicalization of a social phenomenon can be driven by the activities of individuals and self-help groups rather than by the medical profession. This could be construed as a consequence of total medicalization of society but Giddens sees it as an example, 'contra Foucault', of individual agency. Seen from this perspective, the Foucauldian focus on texts and discourse neglects the ways in which doctors and lay people act and leaves no scope for resistance or action. All one is left with are docile bodies. In contrast Lupton emphasizes that power is a relational thing and resistance is everywhere. The lay experience of the 'phenomenological body' as she calls it is absent from 'orthodox' Foucauldian accounts. She argues that the relationship between clinicians and patients is much more ambivalent and contingent than some Foucauldian researchers might suggest. Patients need to trust health professionals at certain times, and this involves a partial surrender of autonomy. At other times the relationship involves a negotiation of power. Lupton does not turn away from Foucault, however, arguing instead that these difficulties might be overcome by Foucault's focus on the technologies of the self. Earlier in this chapter I suggested that Foucault's view of the self was limited. It seems to me that his idea of a 'self-created self' falls back into an asocial idea of the self.

In contrast to Foucault, Habermas' work seems under-utilized in relation to medicalization. Links can be made to medicine's role in the colonization of the lifeworld and the distortions of communication that result from medical expertise and medical domination. Habermas draws a distinction between 'purposive-rational' action and 'communicative' action. The former is a technical rationality embedded in social systems such as welfare systems and in markets. The latter is a form of linguistic interaction aimed at achieving understanding. The paradox of rationality is found in the way that social systems colonize the 'lifeworld' (where social interaction and culture are sustained and reproduced) with rationality that has positive and negative characteristics and effects (Thompson, 1984). This analysis is relevant to medicine because of the ways in which medical expertise mediates the colonization of the lifeworld. Medical expertise earns social respect and kudos on the basis of formal knowledge which presents itself as 'purposive-rational' action (Friedson, 1986). This has positive consequences because medicine makes important contributions towards the meeting of generalizable interests. It also has negative consequences through the use of formal knowledge to legitimate the vested interests of the powerful. Medicine's place in the world is contradictory precisely because it has a claim to being hugely beneficial to society and because it plays a major role in the systemizing tendencies of late modernity (Porter, 1998). However, in advanced capitalism there is a tendency towards systematically distorted communication. Public debate is continually distorted by manipulation and powerful media influences. This can lead to frustration and an increasing pessimism as debates seem to become dominated by experts. The technical demands of discourse in high modernity leads to terminological requirements that are beyond the scope of the general populace and restrict debate to those who are capable of using the accepted technical vocabularies. At the same time politicians and policy makers draw on the language of the lifeworld to legitimate further systemization while inventing new arcane, vague, ambiguous and deliberately confusing means of presenting the consequences of their policies back to the general public. The new genetics and allied technology have allowed, and will allow, medicine to probe bodies in greater depth than ever before. These advances bring with them a gaze that expands the capacity to diagnose illness and the risk of future illness. Often this is without any prospect of there being any appropriate treatment. This, I suggest, takes medicalization into a new form, for the success of medicine is in its predictive/diagnostic capacity, throwing an increasing number of people into the category of being ill or about to be ill without the means to cure. These trends have the capacity to expand and deepen the role of medicine in the political and technical control of individuals. Beck (1992) sees these trends as enhancing the social power of the medical profession through the global market for new technologies. But we need to be able to move beyond the rather bland statement that the new genetics is extending the clinical gaze deeper into bodies and communities to consider the ways in which individuals and groups in society interact with these scientific developments.

Globalization and health

Today, everyone is affected by processes of globalization that operate in complex and contradictory ways in a variety of fields from the economic to the political to the cultural. It is possible to overstate the depth of globalization as well as the powerlessness of individuals and governments to address its dangers. However, the vast volume of economic exchange at a global level and the ability of capital to move around the globe almost instantaneously should leave us in no doubt that its effects are all-pervasive and, most importantly, *uneven* (Giddens, 1999). The uneven effects of globalization have been most vividly portrayed by Zigmund Bauman (1998), who uses the terms 'tourists' and 'vagabonds' to illustrate the polarization that accompanies globalization. He outlines the condition of the global elites and the global poor and discusses numerous parallels and dichotomies in their experiences and conditions. Polarization is connected to consumption and mobility. Whereas the global elites are perpetually mobile and indulge in an aesthetics of consumption and extravagant displays of spending, the poor are failed consumers characterized by an immobility, a rootedness. Like Victorian street children with their faces pressed up against a sweet shop window their failure is brought home to them because the global media and communications industry allow them daily viewing of the displays of wealth and consumption. The local and the global are therefore profoundly linked in a myriad of ways, prompting Robertson to talk of 'glocalization' (Robertson, 1994). The consequences for our understanding of health and medicine are profound and can be illustrated by reference to the globalization of health-related industries and the shifting of responsibility for health and social protection back on to the individual. For example, in their review of the pharmaceutical industry, Tarabusic and Vickery (1998) show how international mergers and acquisitions, and joint ventures have proliferated during the last twenty years. These developments allowed pharmaceutical firms to develop links in biotechnology, R&D and to consolidate market positions. The necessity for firms to have a presence in foreign markets means that for most countries pharmaceutical supplies are managed by foreign-controlled firms, with the USA at the centre of this web of global markets. Government policies are very important for an industry that is heavily regulated by polices that address health and safety, intellectual property rights, and trade and competitions policies. The profit margins of the industry are determined by the relationship between R&D costs and the time frame of trials and licence procedures for new drugs and technologies. Protection of patents is an important way of protecting profits for the industry and there is an increasing global pressure to favour company needs over consumer welfare. This is just one example of the ways in which healthcare systems are becoming increasingly globalized and systematized. And, one of the driving forces behind this systemization is the asymmetrical relationship between consumerism in the developed world and productivism in the developing world.

Noam Chomsky (1998) has highlighted the threats to democracy from the Multilateral Agreement on Investment (MAI) and has charted the involvement of powerful corporate interests in battles over the MAI with grass-roots organizations. Habermas' ideas concerning a deliberative democracy on a global scale may offer a means of extending this critique. His response lies with the notion of law as a medium of communicative practices, but here he is open to the charge of naïvety and Occidentalism, forever in danger of reinforcing the power of global elites. Given the devastating impact of processes of globalization on world health (Navaroo, 1999), Habermas can be criticized for not addressing the problem of unequal power relations in advanced capitalism (Callanicos, 1999). I would suggest that while his analysis takes us further than any Foucauldian account of power, it needs to be tempered by Chomsky's comment that 'answers are not determined by words, but by the power relations that impose their interpretations' (Chomsky, 1998: 26).

Surveillance and governmentality

Foucault has had a profound influence over sociological thought through his work on governmentality (Foucault, 1991). Power cannot just be seen as embedded in the state or in institutions, it is constituted in social relations, and governance therefore is the regulation of society not by the state but by its own structures. The era of high modernity is one that is characterized by an endemic crisis of welfare which has brought with it a number of social transformations, not least of which is the increasing emphasis given to individual responsibility. New dilemmas and anxieties arise from an ever-expanding multiplicity of choices (Bauman, 1998) and new-found freedoms have a sting in their tail as they require us to choose carefully in the face of calculable and incalculable risks. For Bauman morality is an existential condition where morality is defined as responsibility for the other, but responsibility entails choice and choices are multiple, ever present, and their conse-quences are ambivalent. Choice has become a burden for individuals. No longer is this burden shouldered by religious forces as in traditional societies or through a hierarchy of authorities and institutions as in modern societies. The focus on the individual today leaves us alone with our choices, facing a plurality of choice and a cacophony of authority and opinion. Ulrich Beck (1992) uses the term 'flexible modernization' to refer to these processes of indi-vidualization.

Castel (1991) has identified a shift in the preventative strategies of public welfare provision from dangerousness to risk, from surveillance to governmentality, and chartered its consequences for medicine and public health. This leads to an expansion of surveil-lance as new risks are continuously manufactured through probability and statistical calculation. David Armstrong has spoken of an extension of the medical gaze into communities through the expansion of public health surveillance (Armstrong, 1995). But this seems to overstate the extent to which surveillance is becoming more intense and universal (Porter, 1996). Governmentality on the other hand (the conduct of conduct) is a space between self-regulation based around technologies of the self and regulation/domination. Its importance for our understanding of the modern state is that the state no longer coerces or dominates but acts in ways that try to direct free will. The state urges people to behave in ways that develop technologies of the self. In this way the state is said to be benign not coercive. Higgs (1998) has linked this to Giddens' identification of the 'disembedding tendency in late modernity'. The negative effect this has on ontological security, Giddens (1994) argues, can be addressed through narratives of the self. It is possible to discern increasing investment by governments in strategies that mix traditional interventions with governmentality (Social Exclusion Unit, 2000). These strategies, however, are likely to be based on the identification of deviations from a frame of reference based on statistical norms and expert-based concepts of normality. Welfare states therefore are increasingly taking assessment and administration as their main function and reducing their interventionist role to one of guidance. Monitoring seems increasingly focused on the goal of identifying risky groups (defined as those incapable of self-surveillance or co-surveillance) and these 'failures' are targeted for more coercive/regulatory interventions. This is based on a growing consensus around modes of behaviour, a consensus that is characterized by its asymmetry, featuring increasing duties and obligations and decreasing collective rights.

There may be other ways of seeing these developments, particularly in the focus on the relationship between our understanding of surveillance and risk. Bauman (1998) revisited panopticism, arguing that it is no longer relevant to our present condition. The panopticon represented modernity, state-adminis-tered surveillance, supra-local integration and normalization, and asymmetrical surveillance. This was particularly useful in its appli-cation to prisons, asylums, hospitals, mass armies and industrial plants. But Bauman sees modern surveillance methods and databases not as devices to ensnare but as a means to categorize, divide and exclude. More importantly he sees a different form of asymmetry in surveillance. He refers to Mathiesen's (1997) 'Synopticon' as a global phenomenon where we are united in the act of watching not being watched, and to Poster's (1996) 'Superpanopticon' which may be more relevant to today's condition, recognizing as it does a collusion with surveillance. We are not forced into being watched, we are seduced into watching, and this seduction reinforces stratifications and inequalities that are taking on new and extreme forms (Young, 1999). These inequalities are particularly relevant to the role of public health, but it is not clear whether public health policies, of themselves, can provide an adequate response. Foucault's critique of normative science is useful here but it seems to me that Habermas' work on participatory and discursive democracy can offer an understanding of the consequences of systematic change for individual health and autonomy.

Conclusion

In this brief account of the work of Habermas and Foucault I have tried to identify the correspondences in their work as well as the differences between them. Habermas sees the exchange of illocutionary speech acts as the means to achieving mutual understanding and consensus. Foucault views consensus as part of the exercise of power. The problem here, as Fraser (1994) points out, is that Foucault calls so many things power. Ultimately this makes a critical position untenable. Habermas, on the other hand, has attempted to reconstruct a universal morality based on formal procedural models of discourse. In doing so he offers opportunities for escaping the conservatism and nihilism of much postmodern thought and may have even prompted some postmodern writers to seek more socially based accounts through arguing for an expansion in democratic and discursive spaces. I began this chapter with two quotations by Habermas and Foucault relating to their views on discourse. In my discussion of medicalization, globalization, and governmentality and surveillance, I hope to have shown how changes in science, in the media and in technology have stimulated the construction of new risks and are altering science's inter-relationship with democracy. These new risks are largely invisible, a characteristic that diminishes the capacity of democratic institutions to respond. We can only extend our understanding of these developments by means of discourse, but to do this I would suggest that we view discourse in terms of intersubjective communication and not as a game.

References

Armstrong, D. (1994) 'Bodies of knowledge and knowledge of bodies'. In Jones, C. and Porter, R. (eds) *Reassessing Foucault: Power, Medicine and the Body (Studies in the Social History of Medicine)*. London: Routledge.
—— (1995) 'The rise of surveillance medicine'. *Sociology of Health and Illness*, 17, 3: 393–404.
Bauman, Z. (1998) *Globalization: The Human Consequences*. Cambridge: Polity Press.

Beck, U. (1992) *Risk Society: Towards a New Modernity*. London: Sage.

Bhaskar, R. (1998) *The Possibility of Naturalism*. London: Routledge.

Bury, M. (1997) *Health and Illness in a Changing Society*. London: Routledge.

Callanicos, A. (1999) *Social Theory: A Historical Introduction*. Cambridge: Polity Press.

Castel, R. (1991) 'From dangerousness to risk'. In Burchell, G., Gordon, C. and Miller, P. (eds) *The Foucault Effect: Studies in Governmentality*. London: Harvester Wheatsheaf.

Chomsky, N. (1998) 'Power in the global arena'. *New Left Review*, 230: 3–27.

Conrad, P. (1999) 'A mirage of genes'. *Sociology of Health and Illness*, 21, 2: 228–41.

Delanty, G. (1999) *Social Theory in a Changing World: Conceptions of Modernity*. Cambridge: Polity Press.

Foucault, M. (1980) *Power/Knowledge: Selected Interviews and Other Writings 1972–1977*. Ed. C. Gordon. Brighton: Harvester.

—— (1984) *The Foucault Reader*. Ed. P. Rabinow. London: Penguin.

—— (1990) *The History of Sexuality, Vol 3: The Care of the Self*. Harmondsworth: Penguin.

—— (1991) 'Governmentality'. In Burchell, R. (ed.) *The Foucault Effect*. Hemel Hempstead: Harvester Wheatsheaf.

Fraser, N. (1989) *Unruly Practices: Power Discourse and Gender in Contemporary Social Theory*. Cambridge: Polity Press.

—— (1994) 'Michel Foucault: a young conservative'. In Kelly, M. (ed.) *Critique and Power: Recasting the Foucault/Habermas Debate*. London: MIT Press.

Friedson, E. (1986) *Professional Powers. A Study of the Institutionalisation of Formal Knowledge*. Chicago, IL: University of Chicago Press.

Giddens, A. (1982) *Profiles and Critiques in Social Theory*. London: Macmillan.

—— (1992) *The Transformation of Intimacy: Sexuality, Love, and Eroticism in Modern Societies*. Cambridge: Polity Press.

—— (1994) *Beyond Left and Right*. Cambridge: Polity Press.

—— (1999) *Globalisation*. Lecture 1 of the Reith Lectures. http:/www.lse.ac.uk/Giddens/reith_99/week1/lecture1.htm

Habermas, J. (1985) *The Philosophical Discourse of Modernity*. Cambridge: Polity Press.

—— (1990) *Moral Consciousness and Communicative Action*. Cambridge: Polity Press.

—— (1996) *Between Facts and Norms: Contributions to a Discourse Theory of Law and Democracy*. Cambridge: Polity Press.

—— (1999) 'The European nation state and the pressures of globalization'. *New Left Review*, 235: 46–59.

Higgs, P. (1998) 'Risk, governmentality and the reconceptualization of citizenship'. In Scambler, G. and Higgs, P. (eds) *Modernity, Medicine and Health*. London: Routledge.

Hoy, D.C. (1998) 'Foucault and critical theory'. In Moss, J. (ed.) *The Later Foucault*. London: Sage.

Illich, I. (1976) *Limits to Medicine. Medical Nemesis: The Expropriation of Health*. Harmondsworth: Pelican.

Kelly, M. (1994) *Critique and Power: Recasting the Foucault/Habermas Debate*. London: MIT Press.

Lupton, D. (1994) *Medicine as Culture, Illness, Disease and the Body in Western Societies*. London: Sage.

—— (1995) *The Imperative of Health, Public Health and the Regulated Body*. London: Sage.

—— (1997) 'Foucault, and the medicalization critique'. In Petersen, A. and Bunton, R. (eds) *Foucault Health and Medicine*. London: Routledge.

Mathiesen, T. (1997) 'The viewer society: Michel Foucault's "Panopticon" revisited'. *Theoretical Criminology*, 1, 2: 215–34.

McCarthy, T. (1994) 'The critique of impure reason: Foucault and the Frankfurt School'. In Kelly, M. (ed.) *Critique and Power: Recasting the Foucault/Habermas Debate*. Cambridge, MA: MIT Press.

Navaroo, V. (1999) 'Health and equity in the world in the era of "Globalisation"'. *International Journal of Health Services*, 29, 2: 215–26.

Nettleton, S. (1989) 'Power and pain: the location of pain and fear in dentistry and the creation of a dental subject'. *Social Science and Medicine*, 29: 1183–90.

Nicholson, L. and Seidman, S. (1995) *Social Postmodernism: Beyond Identity Politics*. Cambridge: Polity Press.

Petersen, A. (1997) 'Risk, governance and the new public health'. In Petersen, A. and Bunton, R. (eds) *Foucault, Health and Medicine*. London: Routledge.

Philip, M. (1990) 'Michel Foucault'. In Skinner, Q. (ed.) *The Return of Grand Theory in the Human Sciences*. Cambridge: Canto; first published 1985.

Porter, R. (1998) *The Greatest Benefit to Mankind: A Medical History of Humanity from Antiquity to the Present*. London: HarperCollins.

Porter, S. (1996) 'Contra-Foucault: soldiers, nurses and power'. *Sociology*, 30, 1: 59–78.

Poster, M. (1996) 'Database as discourse, or electronic interpellations'. In Heelas, P., Lash, S. and Morris, P. (eds) *Detraditionalization*. Oxford: Blackwell.

Reinicke, W.H. (1998) *Global Public Policy, Governing Without Government?* Washington: Brookings Institution Press.

Robertson, R. (1994) 'Globalization or glocalization'. *Journal of International Communications*: 1.

Smart, B. (1998) 'Foucault, Levinas and the subject of responsibility'. In Moss, J. (ed.) *The Later Foucault*. London: Sage.

Social Exclusion Unit (2000) *National Strategy for Neighbourhood Renewal: A Framework for Consultation*. London: Cabinet Office.

Tarabusic, C.C. and Vickery, G. (1998) 'Globalization in the pharmaceutical industry. Part II'. *International Journal of Health Services*, 28, 2: 281–303.

Thompson, J. (1984) 'Rationality and social rationalization: an assessment of Habermas' theory of communicative action'. In Thompson, J. (ed.) *Studies in the Theory of Ideology*. Cambridge: Polity Press.

White, S. (1997) 'Not always suffered, but sometimes enjoyed: power contra-Porter'. *Sociology*, 31, 2: 347–51.

Young, J. (1999) *The Exclusive Society*. London: Sage.

Chapter 9

Civil society, the public sphere and deliberative democracy

Graham Scambler and Leslie Martin

The concept of 'civil society' has attracted renewed interest of late as sociologists and others struggle to come to terms with what many take to be novel and vigorous processes of social change. The largely unexpected events of 1989 in eastern Europe, for example, occasioned many to ponder the possible contributions to change fashioned in the apparently re-politicized and revitalized civil societies of nations long accustomed to authoritarian socialism (Arato, 1993). But it remains a concept more enthusiastically invoked than defined. Moreover it undeniably has a rhetorical ring to it (Seligman, 1992). Certainly as opinions on its usefulness or otherwise have proliferated over the last decade they have become more polarized. Hall (1995: 25) is among those with an unapologetically positive view of civil society: 'civil society is a particular form of society, appreciating social diversity and able to limit the depredations of political power, that was born in Europe; it may, with luck, skill and imagination, spread to some other regions of the world'. Hann (1996: 1) takes an entirely different line in his introduction to a collection of anthropological papers which challenge 'western models' of civil society, insisting that 'the term is riddled with contradictions and the current vogue predicated on a fundamental ethnocentricity'.

This chapter is by no means unusual in attributing considerable – and on the whole positive – significance to the concept of civil society, but it is perhaps unusual in its approach. In the first section there is a focused discussion of the related notions of civil society and the public sphere. A new conceptualization of the links between civil society and the private and public spheres of the lifeworld is proffered at this point. The second section introduces and attributes importance to what is often referred to as 'deliberative democracy'. The third section reflects on the relevance of social movements for the establishment and practice of deliberative democracy. And in the fourth and final section the relationships between an effective critical sociology, civil society, the public sphere and deliberative democracy are explored.

Civil society and the public sphere

Defining civil society

Civil society has conventionally been distinguished from the apparatus of the state (Ehrenberg, 1999). Habermas, and others who have developed his perspective, have come to distinguish it too from the economy (see Cohen and Arato, 1992). For Habermas (1996) civil society exists at the interface of the private and public spheres of the lifeworld. It consists of those 'more or less spontaneously emergent associations, organizations and movements that, attuned to how societal problems resonate in the private life spheres, distil and transmit such reactions in amplified form to the public sphere' (Habermas, 1996: 367). It is suggested here that it may be both useful and appropriate to distinguish between two 'sectors' of civil society. What we shall call the *enabling sector* of civil society is located in, or derives its impetus from, the private sphere. It is within the enabling sector that – as part and parcel of the ordinary everyday intercourse of the lifeworld (and typically in what Oldenburg (1997) has helpfully analysed as informal meeting, or 'third', places) – issues of potential concern arise and are often identified. The *protest sector* of civil society is located in, or is directed towards, the public sphere. It is within the protest sector that people come together, or are mobilized, in networks, campaign groups, social movements and other forms of association in pursuit of influence for purposeful change (third places are often important here too).

To return to Habermas, the core of civil society, or what we have called its protest sector, comprises a network of associations that institutionalize 'problem-solving discourses on questions of general interest': 'these *discursive designs* have an egalitarian, open form of organization that mirrors essential features of the kind of communication around which they crystallize and to which they lend continuity and permanence' (original emphasis). It is axiomatic that civil society affords a limited scope for action. Moreover, a robust civil society can only develop in a 'liberal' political culture; its actors can acquire influence, but not political power; and the effectiveness of politics is in any event severely constrained in modern – functionally differentiated – societies. Civil society is 'no macrosubject' able to 'bring society as a whole under control and simultaneously act for it' (Habermas, 1996: 372). Nevertheless, Habermas does submit that the social movements, citizen initiatives and forums, political and other group associations that make up civil society can 'under certain circumstances' acquire influence in the public sphere which extends to the political domain.

The rise and putative fall of the 'bourgeois public sphere'

Habermas' (1989) account of the emergence and changing nature of the public sphere is well known. He argues that a 'bourgeois public sphere' first emerged in eighteenth-century England (and shortly after in other European nations). It was not part of the state but, on the contrary, a sphere in which activities of the state could be confronted and subjected to criticism. 'The medium of this confrontation was itself significant: it was the public use of reason, as articulated by private individuals engaged in argument that was *in principle* open and unconstrained' (Thompson, 1993: 176; original emphasis). The development of the English bourgeois public sphere was facilitated by the rise, first, of the periodical press – including the *Tatler*, the *Spectator*, Defoe's *Review* and Swift's *Examiner* – and second, of a variety of new 'centres of sociability', third, places like salons and coffee houses, in towns and cities. Censorship and political control were also more relaxed than in other parts of Europe. Habermas maintains that the critical discussion engendered in the public sphere gradually led to an opening up and scrutinizing of Parliament, which abandoned its right to prevent publication of its proceedings, and to the constitutional extension of rights of freedom of speech and expression. But according to Habermas the bourgeois public sphere was to experience a fairly rapid decline or 're-feudalization'. The state became more 'capitalist' and more interventionist. At the same time the salons and coffee houses declined and the periodicals were absorbed into an increasingly commercialized system of mass communications (Webster, 1995). 'What was once an exemplary forum of rational-critical debate became just another domain of cultural consumption, and the bourgeois public sphere collapsed into a sham world of image creation and opinion management in which the diffusion of media products is in the service of vested interests' (Thompson, 1993: 178). This account is not without its critics. Thompson (1995) lists four qualifications, all of which have substance. First, by focusing exclusively on the *bourgeois* public sphere, Habermas neglects salient 'popular' forms of public discourse and activity which were not subsumed by, and were sometimes ardently and militantly opposed to, bourgeois sociability (Negt and Kluge, 1993) (for England, see the work of Thompson (1965) and Hill (1975)). Habermas (1992) has recently acknowledged this deficiency in his original account. Second, while the examples of the periodical press cited by Habermas were undoubtedly influential, there is evidence that many of their predecessors were no less so, notably at the time of the English Civil War. Third, although Habermas is aware that the bourgeois public sphere was restricted to individuals with education and the material means to participate, he fails to comment adequately on the fact that it excluded women. The point has been forcibly made that the exclusion of women was *constitutive* of the public sphere: paradigmatically, the public sphere was juxtaposed to the private sphere in a gender-specific way. Habermas has since accepted this criticism too, but perhaps without yet thinking through its ramifications for his own position. And fourth, the view that the bourgeois public sphere went into precipitous decline has been challenged. Thompson (1995), for instance, contends that Habermas overstates the passivity of 'recipients of media products'. He criticizes him too for referring to the re-feudalization of the public sphere, suggesting that, however understandable such a description may be:

> we need to think again about what 'publicness' means today in a world permeated by new forms of communication and information diffusion, where individuals are able to interact with others and observe persons and events without ever encountering them in the same spatio-temporal locale.
>
> (Thompson, 1995: 75)

All four criticisms are telling against Habermas' original account, since revised in some crucial respects (Habermas, 1992, 1996); and the last is especially pertinent to a consideration of the nature of the public sphere in the late twentieth century. There are, in fact, many who share Habermas' pessimism, whatever dissensus may remain on its articulation. Barber (1996: 269) unsurprisingly forbears to write of a re-feudalization of the public sphere in the USA, but he does refer to 'the literal vanishing of civil society', which he distinguishes from both state and economy. Interestingly, he links what he regards as the demise of civil society – complete with its capacity to mediate between state and economy – with the increasingly polarized debate taking place in the USA and elsewhere between communitarians and liberals or individualists. Other commentators have attributed what they too perceive as a diminution and damaging of civil society and the public sphere to the impact of rapidly evolving and highly commercialized mass media and information technologies, many referring specifically to television (for a discussion, see Dahlgren, 1995). Mayhew (1997) has volunteered a related thesis, namely, that professional specialists, using market and promotional campaigns, have come to dominate public communication. He writes of a 'New Public', subject to mass persuasion through relentless advertising, lobbying and other forms of media manipulation.

Others, with varying degrees of affinity with his critical theoretical programme, have addressed the challenge laid down by Habermas, and by those like Thompson who are reluctant to focus exclusively on the *anti-democratic* potential of the new globalizing, increasingly ubiquitous – and 'colonizing' – technologies of communication, to devise means to facilitate and institutionalize discourse-ethical procedures, or the public use of reason, in the public sphere. It is in this context that commentators have come to refer to 'discursive' or 'deliberative' democracy.

Deliberative democracy

Deliberative democracy in principle

There are now a number of philosophical defences of deliberative democracy, not all of them dealing with the same concept (see Bohman and Rehg, 1997). Drawing on his discourse ethics, Habermas (1996, 1998) has recently sought to analyse the phenomena of law and democracy, offering in the process a defence of a proceduralist concept of deliberative democracy in which the burden of legitimating state power is borne by informal and legally institutionalized processes of political deliberation (Cronin and De Greiff, 1998). Of fundamental importance here is the idea that the legitimacy of political authority can only be secured through public participation in political deliberation and decision making; he claims, in fact, that there is an internal relation between the rule of law and popular sovereignty. One way of understanding this is to see Habermas as taking what is valuable and acceptable from each of two contrasting and otherwise fallacious approaches, 'liberalism' and 'communitarianism'.

Habermas defines liberalism as focusing principally on 'autonomy', and communitarianism on 'legitimacy'. Both approaches hold that basic legal and political principles must be morally grounded: liberalism emphasizes individual liberty, while communitarianism emphasizes the values emergent in particular religious, ethnic or national identities, which are transmitted culturally and which form the background against which all questions of political justice must be answered. Habermas opposes this assumption that the law requires to be morally grounded, contending instead that the law and morality stand in a 'complementary relation': the core human rights enshrined in the law are, he asserts, *legal* and not moral rights. He asks which core rights free and equal citizens must confer on one another if they are to organize their affairs through positive law. These fall, he suggests, into five categories: the first three rights – those membership rights and due-process rights that together guarantee private autonomy – constitute the 'negative liberties'; the fourth are rights of political participation and guarantee public autonomy; and the fifth are social-welfare rights, necessary in so far as the effective exercise of civil and political rights depends on citizens being able to satisfy certain basic material needs.

The power of the state is necessary to police this system of rights, which for Habermas introduces a tension between state power and legitimate law. He argues that an account of the public use of reason is essential here, and that this must ultimately refer to democratic processes of opinion- and will-formation in the public sphere. Thus he links the informal discursive sources of democracy with the formal decision-making institutions necessary for the effective rule of law in complex modern societies. Democracy, in Delanty's (1999: 88) words, 'mediates between the public sphere (the domain of debate) and the rule of law (the institutional realm)'. Habermas argues that it is the constitutional state that represents the crucial network of legal institutions and mechanisms that governs the conversion of citizens' communicative power into legitimate administrative activity. Law, for him, 'represents ... the medium for transforming communicative power into administrative power' (Habermas, 1996: 169).

The legitimacy of legal norms, then, is a function of those formal properties of procedures of political deliberation and decision making that support the presumption that their outcomes are rational. In practice, Habermas suggests this requires a public sphere characterized by open political discussion, informed by inputs of expert knowledge and delivering ready access to print and electronic media, and institutionally underwritten by the voluntary associations of civil society. This public sphere would need to be supported by a legally regulated government sphere, consisting of legislative, judicial and administrative branches.

Deliberative democracy in practice

Habermas' model has a measure of consistency with the present institutions of a number of constitutional democracies (although his argument concerning the legitimating function of public reason remains original); but what, more tangibly, might deliberative democracy look like and how might it arise? There have been several contributions here from the USA. Barber (1996), for example, has set out nine defining characteristics of deliberative democracy. He summarizes these as follows: 'A public voice – a voice that is common, deliberative, inclusive, provisional, willing to listen and able to learn, rooted in lateral communication and both founded on and encouraging to imagination, and capable of empowering those who speak – is a voice inflected very differently from either the officially univocal voice of government or the obsessively contrary talk of the private sector's multiple special interests' (Barber, 1996: 280). He realizes that progressing towards deliberative democracy involves more than establishing appropriate 'institutions' (as acknowledged in Rehg's (1994) notion of 'concrete rational solidarity'; see also Chambers (1996)); and he makes the point that the institutions necessary to nurture 'an actual public voice' are 'for the most part still to be created' in the USA. Elsewhere, in more speculative and 'experimental' mode, he writes of the need for an 'American civic forum', and considers the assorted properties of local assemblies, national service, the election of assembly members by sortition (by lot, as with jury pools), the civic uses of new technologies and common work. He commends the practices of bodies like American Health Decisions, the Industrial Areas Foundation, the Study Circles Movement, political juries and deliberative video town meetings of the kind pioneered by Fishkin (1991) (see Barber, 1984).

Mayhew (1997) too asks about possible forums for deliberative democracy. He speculates about an 'imaginary institution', a National Citizens' Forum (NCF), established under the aegis of a hypothetical national association, Citizens for Democratic Deliberation (CDD). In practice, CCD would choose a panel of public representatives to interrogate key policy makers, opinion leaders or candidates. Mayhew (1997: 266) accepts the unfeasibility of such an initiative, but suggests that the exercise of 'simply imagining what it would entail will clarify what is meant by the notion of a "redemptive forum"'. Its success, in his view, would depend on the achievement of four conditions. The NCF's 'legiti-macy' would be contingent, first, on both it and CDD being viewed as *impartial*. Panellists would achieve their legitimacy by taking the role of 'prolocutors' for the public. *Publicity* is Mayhew's second condition: without national publicity through the mass media – and, ideally, the simultaneous broadcast of its sessions on all major television networks – the NCF could not achieve its purpose. The third condition is *representation*. Acknowledging that a 'wide range of voices representing diverse perspectives, interests and experi-ences' would need to be included, Mayhew writes of the possibility of establishing local deliberative groups (along the lines of the National Issues Forums); reports could be submitted to the CDD, selected issues treated by the NCF, and the convenors of local groups even coopted to the national panel. The fourth condition is *access to leaders*. Means would have to be found to ensure the coop-eration of 'national leaders': 'NCF would rely on their capacity to create social pressure to cooperate, which in turn would depend on public ratification of the Forum's claim to be acting as prolocutors on behalf of the public' (Mayhew, 1997: 268). Ultimately it would be public ratification that would grant 'influence' to the NCF.

Some observations

A number of general observations concerning civil society, the public sphere, deliberative democracy and their linkages might be made at this juncture. A first point reverts to Habermas' claim that the bourgeois public sphere, associated initially with late-eighteenth-century Europe, had significant progressive properties. This is probably an apposite claim, although the bourgeois public sphere certainly remained, as many feminists have emphasized, a socially restricted and exclusionary dimension of the lifeworld. The question as to whether or not it has since receded is not straightforward. It is as easy to overstate its extent, ubiquity and promise two centuries ago as it is to embrace pessimism now. It is important, however, to resist the temptation – whether communitarian, 'multiculturalist' or postmodern – to prematurely reject the concept of a *single* (formal) public sphere in favour of a multiplicity of (substantive) public spheres (see, for example, Calhoun, 1996), an issue we return to below.

The separation of civil society and the public sphere from the economy as well as the state is vital in modern society, much American analysis notwithstanding (for a discussion, see Harrington Watt, 1991). In his analysis of free speech, Garnham (1992) stresses the unsatisfactory nature of the traditional liberal view that only the market can offset the prospect of state surveillance and coercion. He supports Habermas' theoretical frame: 'Habermas distinguishes the public sphere from both state and market and can pose the question of the threats to democracy and the public discourses upon which it depends coming from the development of an oligopolistic capitalist market and from the development of the modern interventionist welfare state' (Garnham, 1992: 361). Moreover, whatever its precise trajectory from the European Enlightenment to the present, there is no doubting 'current' constraints on actors in civil society and the depth of the penetration or 'colonization' of the public sphere by the media of the marketplace and the state; nor that aspects of system rationalization and lifeworld colonization have exacted costs in terms of, and represent a continuing threat to, democratic accountability and any fledgling potential for deliberative democracy.

There is no gainsaying the existence of 'deliberative inequalities' in the public sphere. Bohman (1996: 110) distinguishes three kinds: *power asymmetries*, which affect access to the public sphere; *communicative inequalities*, which affect the ability to participate and to make effective use of available opportunities to deliberate in the public sphere; and *political poverty*, which makes it unlikely that 'politically impoverished' citizens can participate in the public sphere at all. He argues that deliberation 'without correction for inequalities' will tend inexorably to elitist practice, 'favouring those who have greater cultural resources (such as knowledge and information) and who are more capable of imposing their own interests and values on others in the public arena' (Bohman, 1996: 112). Fraser (1992) suggests that deliberative inequalities might themselves be articulated or 'thematized' in the public sphere. This could involve, for example, 'challenging unfair advantages in the public sphere due to social and economic position; introducing the effects of privately owned and profit-driven media on the circulation of information in discussion; and investigating the way social and economic subordination filters into and distorts the public sphere' (Chambers, 1996: 207).

Finally, while there is self-evidently little cause for optimism about the immanent prospects for enhanced democratic accountability through lifeworld rationalization – and Habermas rightly remains pessimistic when switching his attention from the 'old' class-based to the 'new' social movements as possible agents of such change – it nevertheless seems difficult to exaggerate the importance of devising ways of giving effective voice to the 'public use of reason'. It may perhaps be helpful to illustrate this in a more tangible fashion. The next section, therefore, focuses on the potential role of social movements.

Social movements and the protest sector of civil society

Defining social movements

Definitions of 'social movements' remain varied and contestable (see Diani, 1992; Zirakzadeh, 1997). A reasonable starting point is probably that of della Porta and Diani (1999: 16), who define social movements in terms of four elements: as (1) informal networks, based on (2) shared beliefs and solidarity, which (3) mobilize about conflictual issues, through (4) the frequent use of various forms of protest. Two perspectives in the analysis of social movements remain especially influential in contemporary sociology: *resource mobilization theory* (in the USA) and *new social movement theory* (in Europe). The former can be said to focus on the 'how' questions concerning social movements: how groups emerge, recruit their members, deal with success or failure, and so on (McAdam *et al.*, 1996). Case studies of social movements from this perspective reveal participants as rational actors. Its theorists dwell on resources – in terms of participants, money, political 'savvy', links with other organizations and media attention – available to specific social movement organizations (Soper, 1994); and how the availability and use of these resources determine when a movement forms, its tactical choices and its trajectory. If resource mobilization theory is concerned principally with 'how' questions, new social movement theory is focused on 'why' questions; and it is with new social movements that we are primarily concerned here.

New social movement theorists typically claim that the social movements of the present generation, under disorganized capitalism, are qualitatively different from their predecessors, under organized capitalism (Calhoun, 1993; Eyerman, 1992). They stress that conflict among the industrial classes is of decreasing relevance and that the representation of movements as largely homogeneous subjects is no longer feasible (della Porta and Diani, 1999: 11–12). Writing in the 1980s, Offe (1985) identified a number of properties of new social movements which distinguish them from the old-style 'workers' movements': a critical stance in relation to modernity and progress; decentralized and participatory organizational strutures; a defence of interpersonal solidarity against the giant colonizing bureaucracies; and the reclamation of autonomous spaces, rather than material advantages. New social movements, for Offe, are characterized by 'an open, fluid organization, an inclusive and non-ideological participation, and greater attention to social than to economic transformations' (della Porta and Diani, 1999: 12).

Two theorists who have developed distinctive and influential accounts of new social movements which are pertinent to the argument in this section are Touraine and Melucci. Touraine's views have evolved considerably over the years and, like Habermas, his attentions have turned increasingly to issues of democracy: while Habermas might be said to offer a 'decontextualized discourse ethic', however, Touraine writes of a 'recomposing of the world' around a 're-enchanted politics' and the need for the invention of a 'cultural democracy' (Delanty, 1999: 138; see Touraine, 1997). As far as social movements are concerned, Touraine has maintained that a society's social movements are found to centre around a 'core conflict' within that society. In the period of organized capitalism, for example, the core conflict arose out of the mode of production and class struggle emerged as the key contest, giving rise to the labour movement. With reference to the present period of disorganized capitalism, Touraine draws a dividing line between a 'logic of the marketplace', also a logic of power and accumulation, and a 'logic of individual liberty', which, he insists, cannot be 'reduced to the affirmation of a self-destructive narcissism, nor to the return to cultural and ethnic roots in which the individual is suppressed in favour of a return to religions and theocracy' (Touraine, 1992: 141). For Touraine, the core conflict in the kind of technocratic or 'programmed' society characteristic of disorganized capitalism might best be described as between technology and the 'bureaucratic control of everyday life' on the one hand, and those who oppose this control on the other. Protest activities unrelated to this core conflict are more appropriately termed 'submovements, communitarian movements, national movements' and so on, and should be considered as subordinate to the core conflict (Diani, 1992: 7). While Touraine once accorded social movements a potential to transform society, he has more recently come to stress the 'plural character' of the new social movements, associating them with democracy and the rights of the individual in the face of encroaching political power.

Melucci (1989, 1994), for whom culture and democracy are also fundamental themes, focuses rather on individuals participating in social movements *qua* 'actors within the limits and possibilities thrown up by structures', emphasizing the need to know how people become involved in collective action, how they construct collective identity and unity, and the meanings produced as a result of this collective work. He introduces the notion of 'submerged networks', contending that social movements do much of their identity creation and subversion of cultural codes while not actually engaged in public protest, but during phases of 'latency'. His own studies of social movements purport to demonstrate that their submerged networks can 'render power visible', even in previously uncontested areas (Mayer and Roth, 1995: 305). His emphasis, then, is on the transmutation of individual identity to collective identity, on the cultural work of social movements, and on conflict. He writes of the importance of 'meaning' in terms of the creation of new cultural codes: 'what lies at the core of contemporary conflicts is the production and reappropriation of meaning' (Melucci, 1996: 145). Social movement activity, for Melucci, moves in and out of the political realm, and it is the processes through which a social movement's participants generate collective identity and act on it, paradigmatically initiating change through the subversion of extant cultural codes and genesis of novel successors, which are of principal importance.

It may be helpful at this point to reflect briefly on the properties of a particular 'sample' network of AIDS activists in the American health domain, *ACT UP*, and to ask whether or not this might reasonably be said to constitute a (new) social movement. *ACT UP*, or 'the AIDS Coalition to Unleash Power', involves a diverse non-partisan group of individuals, united in anger and committed to using direct action to end the AIDS crisis (see Halcli, 1999). This 'welcome', given at *ACT UP* meetings across the USA, indicates that participants are united by a clear cause, and suggests that they come from varied backgrounds to contribute. In reality, however, the majority of *ACT UP* participants have proved to be young, white, gay males who have previous experience as activists (Elbaz, 1995). The ethnic and gender diversity of 'chapters' seems to relate to the willingness of the chapter to acknowledge the irreducible oppression and experiences of people of colour and of women, as well as of others like drug users. Several *ACT UP* groups have in fact splintered over the past decade over just this issue, that is, over whether or not *ACT UP*'s policy should be to actively confront racism, sexism and so on.

The organizational structure of *ACT UP* resonates with standard accounts of new social movements. Each chapter is loosely affiliated with the national network and works on any issues local participants judge relevant. There is no hierarchical leadership structure, or indeed formal membership, and group decisions are usually reached by consensus. *ACT UP* works on several levels: its members engage in specific strategic actions, such as demanding a reduction in drug prices; symbolic protests, for example utilizing stickers and posters showing bloody hands to proclaim that the Reagan administration had blood on its hands because of its protracted inaction in the face of the AIDS epidemic; and ongoing projects to subvert cultural codes and images, like disavowing the 'innocent/guilty' dichotomy, popularizing the SILENCE=DEATH symbol, and the literal subversion of the pink triangle used to identify homosexuals during the Holocaust. *ACT UP* is of course not alone in this work. Jennes (1993) has described the efforts of *COYOTE* (Call Off Your Tired Old Ethics), a prostitutes' rights organization in the USA, to combat the image of sex workers as 'vectors of disease'. And similar battles are waged by gay, Haitian and drug-using groups. Over the two decades of the AIDS crisis, in fact, there has been substantial cooperation between such groups; the need for large numbers of activists to push for change, and the recognition of common plights and agendas, have led to a high degree of networking among these communities.

Does *ACT UP* conform to the criteria for a social movement advanced by della Porta and Diani? It seems that it does, and that it is in fact reasonable to regard *ACT UP* as a new social movement. It is certainly, first, an informal network. And no less certainly, second, its activists demonstrate shared beliefs and solidarity, possibly a reaction to their early portrayal as social pariahs. This sense of identification remains strong, despite the fact that the diagnosis of HIV/AIDS has become less stigmatizing through the 1990s. Although short of the numbers and high degree of network coordination found in, say, the US Civil Rights movement, AIDS activists have continued to pull together a wide range of supporters for such actions as national phone 'zaps' around drug approval and marches on Washington in favour of needle exchange. In fact, collective action on conflictual issues, third, is perhaps the strongest feature of *ACT UP*'s endeavours. AIDS activists necessarily advocate positions contrary to 'traditional' American sensibilities: for example, on issues of sex, sexuality, drug use, condom distribution in schools, health care for all regardless of ability to pay and the confidentiality of all medical records. Such positions and demands are non-negotiable, and even if incrementalism is tolerated for a while they are not abandoned. Protests, fourth, remain an indispensable part of these activists' armoury.

Two aspects of Melucci's account of new social movements are especially relevant to *ACT UP*'s activities. His perspective on how individuals become part of a movement, how movement identity is created, and what this sense of collective identity means to and for participants, cannot be properly applied here, but even a cursory analysis of *ACT UP*'s recurring themes, slogans and symbols is suggestive. AIDS is a life and death issue, and this provides the basis for much of AIDS activists' sense of collective identity. The other side of SILENCE=DEATH is ACTION=LIFE. The symbolic value of activism is revealed here: 'We die, you do nothing' is a common theme at 'die-ins', drawing a sharp boundary between activists and 'non-active others'. These chants and symbols show the active creation of a salient collective identity. Melucci is also interested in periods of latency in social movements. The election of a Democratic president, the appointment of a federal 'AIDS czar' and the discovery of promising AIDS treatments have all served to dampen some of the fire previously displayed by activists. Activists still exist, but are working on more subtle issues and using less visible tactics. If *ACT UP* emerges intact from this current period, this will lend support to Melucci's conception of 'submerged networks', as well as to the definition of AIDS activism as a social movement.

Touraine's stringent, less compromising definition of a social movement, that is, as centred on the 'core conflict' of disorganized capitalism, seems more difficult to reconcile with *ACT UP* and AIDS activism. The immediate and original goals of AIDS activists, namely, ready access to treatments, accurate prevention information and an end to discrimination against people living with HIV/AIDS, do not appear to be in line with Touraine's core conflict. It might perhaps be argued that the ideals behind these immediate pragmatic issues, together with the more general goals of health care for all and freedom from social prejudice against drug users and sex workers, as well as, more generally, from homophobia, racism and sexism, are not inconsistent with Touraine's contemporary core conflict of the individual versus the repressive, bureaucratic or programmed society; but – for the time being at least – these broader social issues remain subsidiary to activists' identification of the more direct needs associated with the AIDS crisis.

(New) social movements and deliberative democracy

In light of the theorization of social movements in general, and of new social movements in particular, and of studies of initiatives like *ACT UP* in the USA, three points might usefully be made concerning linkages between social movements, the protest sector of civil society, the public sphere of the lifeworld, and deliberative democracy. The first point is that many of the social movements emergent in the protest sector of civil society in disorganized capitalism – like *ACT UP* for example – not only serve as 'carriers' of communicative rationality into the public sphere, but also typically possess organizational and other properties which are suggestive of, or even qualify them as prototypes for, deliberative democracy (Habermas, 1996). Moreover, as Bohman (1996) notes, they can have a significant impact on deliberative inequalities. He writes of this type of social movement:

> First, it is a mechanism for pooling the resources, capacities and experiences of various persons and groups, and it gives coherent expression and unified voice to their shared problems and grievances. Second, solidarity within these informal networks permits pooling of resources and information and thus the creation of public goods within the movement as a way to compensate for resource inequalities and political poverty. The organization of the movement itself also gives it a voice, putting it in dialogue with other actors and institutions who recognize their grievances as public problems or expand the pool of their public reasons. Small acts of contestation can then be generalized into protests and become a public challenge to the existing distribution of deliberative resources in institutions. Once given powerful public expression, the movement's grievances can be publicly recognized as legitimate and made part of the public agenda for decision-making institutions.
>
> (Bohman, 1996: 137)

Second, it is too readily assumed that the putative demise of the old labour movements of organized capitalism signals the end of the era of 'revolutionary politics' and aspirations. Disorganized capitalism is associated in most commentators' minds not only with the new social movements but with a more modest 'post-revolutionary politics'. Habermas (1987) sees new social movements as occupying an ambivalent position as a post-revolutionary radical consciousness and as the sign of a new kind of politics. Delanty (1999: 85) summarizes: 'Habermas assumes that ideology has come to an end and in its place is a "fragmented consciousness". But fragmentation is not seen as something that fundamentally challenges the autonomy of communicative action. It is his thesis that fragmentation results from the colonization of the lifeworld by outside, objective forces emanating from the system. Fragmentation is purely a matter of cognition, an "obscurity" in the late modern condition.'

Hunter (1995) is one who warns against the over-inclusive and premature abandonment of the revolutionary tradition that this entails. He rightly maintains that the post-revolutionary goals of the new social movements can *in fact* only be achieved in the event of radical, even revolutionary, social change. He is worth quoting at some length here:

> Today's social movements set numerous goals that cannot be realized through modest reform. Most revolutionary theory has focused on how revolutions can be made, not on the world they would create, and little agreement exists 'on what constitutes movement success' (Tarrow, 1989). Still, it is possible to specify political goals enunciated by contemporary social movements and underscore the extent of economic, political, and cultural transformation their realization would entail. Economic goals include reducing and then ending hunger, physical deprivation, gross economic inequality, and undemocratic, elite control of material and financial resources. Green social movements focus on stopping environmental degradation and pursuing sustainable development grounded in an ecological critique of industrializing modernity. Identity-based new social movements seek the end of domination and marginality defined by racism, national chauvinism, sexism and homophobia. Peasant-based popular movements fight for land and water and against monoculture agribusiness. Indigenous people seek rights, autonomy, and the preservation of their lands and resources. In addition to these substantive goals, social movements and organizations are struggling for a dramatic invigoration and expansion of democracy, enrichment of civil society and public spheres, extensions of human rights globally, and form commitments to individual freedom from state domination and repressive cultural norms.
>
> (Hunter, 1995: 325)

What this 'brief list' indicates, Hunter (1995: 325) emphasizes, is 'the need for the transformation of broad phenomena – undemocratic political institutions, economic, racial and gender inequities, and industrialism's threats to humans and nature – not "just" the amelioration of particular problems'. In a passage recalling our earlier discussion of *ACT UP*, he writes:

> it may be impossible to achieve a world in which, for instance, diseases like AIDS do not emerge; but its epidemiology would have been very different and much less deadly if Africa were

less impoverished, if billions of dollars were redirected from arms purchases to infrastructural development, if women had more power globally, if homosexuals were not discriminated against, and if sexually represssive ethics did not structure most public discourse about AIDS prevention.

(Hunter, 1995: 325–6)

And third, it has of course to be recognized that there seems little prospect for the foreseeable future of the 'revolutionary' social change required to make the disparate, discrete and *seemingly* straightforward and modest objectives of contemporary social movements attainable in practice. Hunter prudently admits as much. Nor is it apparent that these movements will make anything other than slow progress as bearers of communicative rationality in civil society and the public sphere, although it is our contention that this remains a salient and important role for them. The principal of numerous obstacles to fulfilment of this role by movements, we would maintain, are relations of class (complemented by those of gender and ethnicity), which are as pivotal for today's disorganized as for yesterday's organized capitalism; relatedly, and despite individuals' undeniably acute sense of a 'fragmented consciousness', it would be premature and foolhardy to abandon the concept of ideology. Even old-style class-based labour movements might yet rise from the ashes.

The significance of a critical sociology

One of us (Graham Scambler) has argued in detail elsewhere that critical sociologists are rationally obligated, in line with a recon-structed Enlightenment project, to reflexively pursue the de-colonization and further rationalization of the lifeworld *as their first priority*, and this is of course incompatible with a primary allegiance to system needs (Scambler, 1996). Moreover this commitment to lifeworld rationalization is a *moral* requirement (Scambler, 1998). This argument is constructed in relation to Habermas' (1990, 1993) theory of discourse ethics, which in many ways represents a deepening of his theory of communicative action. It starts from a *principle of universalization* which both echoes and departs from that of Kant: 'the emphasis shifts from what each can will without contradiction to be a universal law to what all can will in agreement to be a universal norm' (McCarthy, 1978: 236). This is to 'socialize' Kant's individualistic moral theory in such a manner as to satisfy objections raised initially by Hegel (see Outhwaite, 1994). Habermas' principle of universalization compels the 'universal exchange of roles' that Mead referred to as 'ideal role taking' or 'universal discourse'. Every valid norm thus has to fulfil the following condition: '*All* affected can accept the consequences and the side-effects its general observance can be anticipated to have for the satisfaction of everyone's interests (and these consequences are preferred to those of known alternative possibilities for regulation)' (Habermas, 1990: 65; original emphasis).

The principle of universalization should not be conflated or confused with the *principle of discourse ethics*, which asserts that 'only those norms can claim to be valid that meet (or could meet) with the approval of all affected in their capacity *as participants in a practical discourse*' (Habermas, 1990: 66; original emphasis). While the principle of universalization has to do with *moral* questions of 'justice' and 'solidarity', which admit of formal resolution, the principle of discourse ethics concerns *ethical* questions about the 'good life', which can only be addressed in the context of substantive cultures, forms of life or individual projects.

Justice and solidarity, to which Habermas accords priority, are necessarily related to, and of the essence of, communicative action. Justice, in its modern sense, refers to the 'subjective freedom of inalienable individuality'; and solidarity refers to the 'well-being of associated members of a community who intersubjectively share the same lifeworld' (Habermas, 1990: 200). Morality, Habermas (1990: 200) insists, 'cannot protect the rights of the individual without also protecting the well-being of the community to which he belongs'. 'Precisely the effort to convince others of the justice of a normative expectation', Rehg (1994: 245) explains, 'demands that I attend empathetically to its effects on others' welfare.'

The moral character of critical sociologists' commitment to lifeworld rationalization also entails a commitment to forums of deliberative democracy via the institutionalization of discourse-ethical procedures in the public sphere of the lifeworld. Their obligation extends also to addressing and publicizing issues of concern in the lifeworld. Meeting this complex and daunting requirement demands a consideration of 'alliances of interest' with other systems and, especially, 'movement intellectuals' and activists in the protest sector of civil society and the public sphere (Eyerman and Jamison, 1991). There are three propositions bearing on this notion of a critical sociology that we would offer by way of a conclusion to this chapter.

The first asserts that there is an *internal relation* – that is, a relation of necessity and moral contiguity or affinity deriving from Habermas' theory of communicative action – between the concepts of 'critical sociology', 'civil society', 'public sphere' and 'deliberative democracy' as explicated and deployed in the course of the arguments of this chapter. It is the nature of this relation that provides the rationale for retaining the notion of a single formal public sphere. While there is no denying either the evidence for multiple substantive working-class and other public spheres emergent alongside the bourgeois public sphere identified by Habermas in England and in other European societies in the eighteenth century, or the existence of a multiplicity of such public spheres in contemporary Britain, neighbouring European nations, the USA and elsewhere, there is in our view a strong and purposeful case for retaining a concept of a single, formal public sphere.

The second proposition clarifies this case. It is that one defining feature of Habermas' concept of a 'public sphere', as of his concept of a 'ideal speech situation', is its *counterfactual status*. Just as the formal concept of an ideal speech situation allows for the substantive identification and investigation of (often colonizing) distortions in 'actually existing' communicative episodes, so the formal concept of a single public sphere allows for the identification and investigation of (often colonizing) distortions in 'actually existing' transnational, national, regional and local public spheres.

The third proposition, linked to the previous two, is that there is a growing obligation and a need on the part of critical sociologists to sponsor the notion of a 'global (critical) sociology'. This, as Martin and Beittel (1998: 139) argue, albeit from a different philosophical vantage point, involves more than extending prevailing research conceptions and agendas, since these are rooted in the comparative method, nationalist practices, and models of European/US development which are 'ill-suited for grasping transnational phenomena and building a worldwide community of sociologists'.

The short- or medium-term prospects for activities within the protest sectors of British or American civil society (informed or otherwise by a critical sociology) leading to a substantive institutionalization of discourse-ethical procedures in the public sphere of the lifeworld – the prospects, that is, for creating deliberative democracy – seem slight indeed. Certainly, as has readily been admitted, the impediments are formidable. For all the prima facie intractability of the problems, however, many of them to do with the exercise of power in narrow sectional system-based interests, the statement of necessary and moral contiguity or affinity between the sociological enterprise and forms of social institutionalization of the *public use of reason* contained in this chapter seems hard to resist, and the consequences of doing so unacceptable. The kind of reflexive critical sociology commended here and supported elsewhere (Scambler, 1996, 1998) cannot but be *radical* (without being partisan), not because it embodies, represents or issues in a particular ethical vision of a 'good society', but precisely because it does not: its intrinsic commitment, necessarily and morally, is 'to' the *public use of reason*, and 'against' any (typically system-driven) impediment – especially Bohman's (1996) 'deliberative inequalities' – to the *public use of reason*.

It is important, finally, to be clear about what is *not* being argued here. It is not being contended that *all* sociologists should become active players or agents in civil society and the public sphere, nor even that they should become critical sociologists in the sense defined here. Sociology is a broad church and much worthwhile endeavour will remain *pre-* or *non-critical*. But it *is* being suggested that sociology *must*, if it is to retain the purpose and impetus of a reconstructed Enlightenment project, best represented currently in the work of Habermas, embody a critical component along the lines sketched here. Sociology, in other words, *must* generate its own 'critical mass' of critical sociologists.

References

Arato, A. (1993) *From Neo-Marxism to Democratic Theory: Essays on the Critical Theory of Soviet-type Societies*. Armonk, NY: M.E. Sharpe.

Barber, B. (1984) *Strong Democracy: Participatory Politics for a New Age*. Berkeley: University of California Press.

—— (1996) 'An American civic forum: civil society between market individuals and the political community'. In Paul, E., Miller, F. and Paul, J. (eds) *The Communitarian Challenge to Liberalism*. Cambridge: Cambridge University Press.

Bohman, J. (1996) *Public Deliberation: Pluralism, Complexity and Democracy*. Cambridge, MA: MIT Press.

Bohman, J. and Rehg, W. (1997) *Deliberative Democracy: Essays on Reason and Politics*. Cambridge, MA: MIT Press.

Calhoun, C. (1993) ' "New" social movements of the early twentieth century'. *Social History*, 17: 385–411.

—— (1996) 'Social theory and the public sphere'. In Turner, B. (ed.) *The Blackwell Companion to Social Theory*. Oxford: Blackwell.

Chambers, S. (1996) *Reasonable Democracy: Jürgen Habermas and the Politics of Discourse*. Ithaca, NY: Cornell University Press.

Cohen, J. and Arato, A. (1992) *Civil Society and Political Theory*. Cambridge, MA: MIT Press.

Cronin, C. and De Greiff, P. (1998) 'Introduction'. In Habermas, J. *The Inclusion of the Other: Studies in Political Theory*. Cambridge: Polity Press.

Dahlgren, P. (1995) *Television and the Public Sphere: Citizenship, Democracy and the Media*. London: Sage.

Delanty, G. (1999) *Social Theory in a Changing World: Conceptions of Modernity*. Cambridge: Polity Press.

della Porta, D. and Diani, M. (1999) *Social Movements: An Introduction*. Oxford: Blackwell.

Diani, M. (1992) 'The concept of social movement'. *Sociological Review*, 92: 1–25.

Ehrenberg, J. (1999) *Civil Society: The Critical History of an Idea*. New York: New York University Press.

Elbaz, G. (1995) 'Beyond anger: the activist construction of the AIDS crisis'. *Social Justice*, 22: 43–76.

Eyerman, R. (1992) 'Modernity and social movements'. In Haferkamp, A. and Smelser, N. (eds) *Social Change and Modernity*. Berkeley: University of California Press.

Eyerman, R. and Jamison, A. (1991) *Social Movements: A Cognitive Approach*. Cambridge: Polity Press.

Fishkin, J. (1991) *Democracy and Deliberation*. New Haven, CT: Yale University Press.

Fraser, N. (1992) 'Rethinking the public sphere: a contribution to the critique of actually existing democracy'. In Calhoun, C. (ed.) *Habermas and the Public Sphere*. Cambridge, MA: MIT Press.

Garnham, N. (1992) 'The media and the public sphere'. In Calhoun, C. (ed.) *Habermas and the Public Sphere*. Cambridge, MA: MIT Press.

Habermas, J. (1987) *The Theory of Communicative Action, Volume Two: Lifeworld and System: A Critique of Functionalist Reason*. Cambridge: Polity Press.

—— (1989) *The Structural Transformation of the Public Sphere: An Inquiry into a Category of Bourgeois Society*. Cambridge: Polity Press.

—— (1990) *Moral Consciousness and Communicative Action*. Cambridge, MA: MIT Press.

—— (1992) 'Further reflections on the public sphere'. In Calhoun, C. (ed.) *Habermas and the Public Sphere*. Cambridge, MA: MIT Press.

—— (1993) *Justification and Application: Remarks on Discourse Ethics.* Cambridge: Polity Press.

—— (1996) *Between Facts and Norms: Contributions to a Discourse Theory of Law and Democracy.* Cambridge: Polity Press.

—— (1998) *The Inclusion of the Other: Studies in Political Theory.* Cambridge: Polity Press.

Halcli, A. (1999) 'AIDS, anger and activism: ACT UP as a social movement organization'. In Freeman, J. and Johnson,V. (eds) *Waves of Protest: Social Movements Since the 1960s.* New York: Rowman & Littlefield.

Hall, J. (1995) 'In search of civil society'. In Hall, J. (ed.) *Civil Society: Theory, History, Comparison.* Cambridge: Polity Press.

Hann, C. (1996) 'Introduction: political society and civil anthropology'. In Hann, C. and Dunn, E. (eds) *Civil Society: Challenging Western Models.* London: Routledge.

Harrington Watt, D. (1991) 'United States: cultural challenges to the voluntary sector'. In Wuthnow, R. (ed.) *Between Markets and States: The Voluntary Sector in Comparative Perspective.* Princeton, NJ: Princeton University Press.

Hill, C. (1975) *The World Turned Upside Down.* Harmondsworth: Penguin.

Hunter, A. (1995) 'Rethinking revolution in light of the new social movements'. In Darnovsky, M., Epstein, B. and Flacks, R. (eds) *Cultural Politics and Social Movements.* Philadelphia, PA: Temple University Press.

Jennes, V. (1993) *Making it Work: The Prostitutes' Rights Movement in Perspective.* New York: Aldine de Gruyter.

Martin, W. and Beittel, M. (1998) 'Toward a global sociology? Evaluating current conceptions, methods and practices'. *The Sociological Quarterly*, 39: 139–61.

Mayer, M & Roth, R (1995) 'New social movements and the transformation to post-fordist society. In eds. Darnovsky, M. Epstein, B & Flacks, R: *Cultural Politics and Social Movements.* Philadelphia; Temple University Press.

Mayhew, L. (1997) *The New Public: Professional Communication and the Means of Social Influence.* Cambridge: Cambridge University Press.

McAdam, D., McCarthy, J. and Zald, M. (1996) *Comparative Perspectives on Social Movements: Political Opportunities, Mobilizing Structures and Cultural Framings.* Cambridge: Cambridge University Press.

McCarthy, T. (1978) *The Critical Theory of Jürgen Habermas.* Cambridge: Polity Press.

Melucci, A. (1989) *Nomads of the Present: Social Movements and Individual Needs in Contemporary Society.* London: Hutchinson Radius.

—— (1994) 'A strange kind of newness: what's "new" in new social movements'. In Larana, E., Johnston, H. and Gusfield, J. (eds) *New Social Movements: From Ideology to Identity.* Philadelphia, PA: Temple University Press.

—— (1996) *The Playing Self: Person and Meaning in the Planetary Age*. Cambridge: Cambridge University Press.

Negt, O. and Kluge, A. (1993) *The Public Sphere and Experience*. Minneapolis: University of Minnesota Press.

Offe, C. (1985) 'New social movements: changing boundaries of the political'. *Social Research*, 52: 817–68.

Oldenburg, R. (1997) *The Great Good Place: Cafés, Shops, Community Centres, Beauty Parlours, General Stores, Bars, Hangouts and How They Get You Through the Day*. New York: Marlowe & Co.

Outhwaite, W. (1994) *Habermas: A Critical Introduction*. Cambridge: Polity Press.

Rehg, W. (1994) *Insight and Solidarity: The Discourse Ethics of Jürgen Habermas*. Berkeley: University of California Press.

Scambler, G. (1996) 'The "project of modernity" and the parameters for a critical sociology: an argument with illustrations from medical sociology'. *Sociology*, 30: 567–81.

—— (1998) 'Medical sociology and modernity: reflections on the public sphere and the roles of intellectuals and social critics'. In Scambler, G. and Higgs, P. (eds) *Modernity, Medicine and Health: Medical Sociology Towards 2000*. London: Routledge.

Seligman, A. (1992) *The Idea of a Civil Society*. New York: Free Press.

Soper, C. (1994) 'Political structures and interest group activism'. *Social Science Journal*, 31: 319–34.

Tarrow, S. (1989) *Struggle, Politics and Reform: Collective Action, Social Movements and Cycles of Protest*. Western Societies Programme Occasional Paper No. 21. Ithaca, NY: Center for International Studies, Cornell University.

Thompson, E. P. (1965) *The Making of the English Working Class*. Harmondsworth: Penguin.

Thompson, J. (1993) 'Review article: the theory of the public sphere'. *Theory, Culture and Society*, 10: 173–89.

—— (1995) *The Media and Modernity: A Social Theory of the Media*. Cambridge: Polity Press.

Touraine, A. (1992) 'Beyond social movements'. *Theory, Culture and Society*, 9: 125–45.

—— (1997) *What is Democracy?* Oxford: Westview Press.

Webster, F. (1995) *Theories of the Information Society*. London: Routledge.

Zirakzadeh, C. (1997) *Social Movements in Politics: A Comparative Study*. London: Longman.

Index